THE THRIVING FAMILY

How to Achieve Home-Life Harmony for You and Your Children

DAVID COLEMAN

HACHETTE
BOOKS
IRELAND

First published in 2012 by Hachette Books Ireland
First published in paperback in 2014 by Hachette Books Ireland
A division of Hachette UK Ltd.

A CIP catalogue record for this title is available from the British Library.

ISBN 9781444726008

Inside design by Sin É Design
Typeset by redrattledesign.com
Cover design by AmpVisual.com
Cover author photo by Ronnie Norton

Printed and bound by CPI Group (UK) Ltd, Croydon, CR0 4YY
Hachette Books Ireland policy is to use papers that are natural, renewable
and recyclable products and made from wood grown in sustainable forests.
The logging and manufacturing processes are expected to conform to the
environmental regulations of the country of origin.

Hachette Books Ireland
8 Castlecourt Centre
Castleknock
Dublin 15, Ireland

A division of Hachette UK Ltd
338 Euston Road
London NW1 3BH
www.hachette.ie

Contents

For My Family

A Note about Family Stories

Throughout the book I have told stories, titled '*A case in point ...*', that illustrate the real-life experiences of families, reflecting a range of situations I have come across in clinical practice. Details such as names, ages and circumstances have been changed in order to protect identities, while giving a genuine account of family life.

01
THE CORE INGREDIENTS FOR A THRIVING FAMILY

Understanding what makes families thrive

The creation of a family is a significant step for any of us to take. When we launch into parenthood, whether planned or unplanned, we carry with us our experiences from our own family upbringing and merge them with our hopes, dreams and aspirations for our children. What an enormous undertaking!

I believe that we want to create the best environment for our children to grow up in so that they can become happy and fulfilled adults. We want our children to thrive, and we work hard to create a safe, structured, nurturing and emotionally rich home life that gives them every opportunity to develop into healthy and independent adults.

We want a family that feels secure and is steady, intimate, connected, understood and thriving. We want a safe reference point for our children to allow them to travel flexibly and resiliently into the world. We want them to be nourished and energised by the time they spend in our family so they can grow and develop and, in time, create their own families. We want them to become responsible members of society, who are capable and dependable, who will make decisions and influence others for good.

If you share these aspirations and goals, this book will help you achieve them.

Hard work and a solid base: the cornerstones of thriving

A colleague once remarked to me that the families who make living look easiest are often those who work hardest. I believe this to be true. We have to invest time and energy in our family and work through good and bad days.

Life is a many-layered experience and some of the issues and dilemmas we face as a family require resilience, determination and a clear set of guiding values to help us navigate the best way forward. Living life according to strong values, like trust, respect, responsibility, honesty, thoughtfulness and kindness, gives us a solid platform to negotiate the ups and downs that come our way.

Thriving families will have strong roots to anchor them in times of uncertainty. They will have the flexibility and resilience to cope with the changing nature of society. Thriving families will feel connected and nurturing to all of their members.

For our families to thrive we must make demands of our children, while simultaneously being responsive to, and considerate of, their needs. Thriving families have high expectations of children and set clear limits about acceptable behaviour. At the same time they offer a warm and approachable atmosphere in which each member can feel accepted and valued. As the adults in a family, we will create this warm but expectant atmosphere.

Effective parenting: the 'kind but firm' approach

Research suggests that the most effective approach to parenting is to show high expectation of our children and their behaviour, with a high level of responsiveness. I like to think of it as kind but firm parenting. Kind, firm parenting is child-centred and typified by warm, nurturing interactions while still setting clear boundaries on children's behaviour. Children who grow up with kind, firm parents tend to be happier, more capable and more successful than others in later life.

It is easy to see why this approach to rearing children is so successful. With a core kindness in place, parents will respond to children breaking limits by forgiving and teaching them, based on the mistake, rather than simply punishing them. Because they are firm, these parents will insist on healthy and helpful rules that keep their children safe and regulate their behaviour.

So, for example, a child might want to go out to meet their friends at 9 p.m. A firm response may be, 'No, you can't go out because it's too late and you have to be up for school tomorrow.' This is likely to be followed up by a thoughtful, understanding (and kind) statement, like, 'You seem disappointed and I guess you may feel you're missing out. Luckily it's Friday tomorrow so you can go out then, but for tonight you have to stay in.'

The effect of authoritarian parenting

Thriving families will always balance demands and expectations with understanding and kindness. The atmosphere in this kind of family is very different from the atmosphere in which only demands and expectations are present. If, for example, we merely make demands of children and have high expectations of them we will probably find that they grow up to be obedient and proficient. They will do what is expected of them, and often to a high standard, but they are less happy and their self-esteem is lower. While they may thrive materially, they won't thrive emotionally.

Firm parents who lack kindness have a high expectation of conformity and compliance from their children. They tend to be restrictive and punitive with a heavy emphasis on limits and rules but without discussion. A typical scenario in such a home would be a parent insisting on hours of music practice, allied to lots of study, with the threat of severe punishment to back up their demands on the children. Giving up the instrument is never an option. At the extreme, many children growing up in these households are fearful and resentful of the power wielded by their parents. This kind of approach meets a parent's need to be in control but is less appropriate to a child's need for warmth, nurturing and understanding.

The effect of kind parenting without firmness

In an environment where parents are responsive to children but place few demands on them, studies show that children tend to be less happy and less able to self-regulate (knowing when to stop eating, when to take rest, and so on). They have greater problems with authority because they are unused to it and typically under-perform at school. Being kind without firmness or setting out expectations of children's behaviour, though in essence nurturing and accepting, problematic because there are no limits, controls or regulation of behaviour. The result is that children may struggle to regulate their behaviour.

In this type of family environment, a child won't necessarily be encouraged to learn an instrument, but if they show interest of their own accord they will be offered lessons. If they then change their mind and choose a new instrument, there will be no problem, with new instruments bought or borrowed, and parents who are delighted that their child is expressing themselves freely. But in a parenting environment that is kind but not firm, the same child might express themselves freely with obstinate refusal to accede to even the most minimal request to be polite, tidy or thoughtful of others. They are learning to be self-centred.

The effect of neither kind nor firm parenting

A more damaging atmosphere still will prevail if parents are neither kind and responsive nor demanding and expectant. At the extreme end of this kind of parenting, parents will be emotionally unsupportive and set no limits on their child's behaviour. As a consequence, these children are more likely to grow up with poor self-control and lower than average self-esteem. Typically they are less competent than their peers since they have never been challenged in the home environment to push themselves, and incidences of truancy from school and general delinquency are more likely.

Our aim, then, is to be kind with our family and to set expectations of them that we will stick to. And, simple as it may seem, these basic tenets of kindness and firmness are all we need to create the best environment for our family to thrive.

This book explores how we can achieve firm but kind parenting.

Determining our values

Our identities will come with us into a new family that we create. The act of creating new life can for many people act as a catalyst to look again at what they value. Most of us know that we will influence the family we create as we were influenced by our parents. When we take on our new role as parent, we must determine what kind of parent we want to be. If we do this consciously we may decide that we want to do things differently from how we were brought up. We might act in different ways and according to new or changed values.

Remembering the past but creating a new future

It helps to be able to consider the different styles of parenting in the context of how we were raised. Most of us will be able to identify the predominant approach our parents took to rearing us. For parents raised in the 1970s and 1980s, a firm, but not necessarily very understanding, approach was the norm. Our parents were products of an even more stridently authoritarian environment where it was the widely accepted view in society that 'children should be seen but not heard'. There was a firmly held intolerance to misbehaviour but little consideration of children's emotional needs.

We may believe that our approach to parenting is 'instinctive', or that we are, in some way, pre-programmed to know how to rear our children. To a certain extent we are, but there are large elements in how we deal with children that are learned. Often we blindly follow the model of how we were parented, or consciously reject that and try to do things differently: the greater our awareness of where we came from and what we do now, the more opportunity we have to do things differently if we want to.

When we try to understand our 'self', most of us can only do it within the context of family. Our families are soldered to our identities. Whatever the constellation of our family of origin (one-parent, two-parent, blended, fostered, adopted or perhaps reared by grandparents), it has insinuated itself into the essence of who we are. Whatever the events, positive or negative, that happened over the course of our childhood or adolescence, our families are central to how we understand or make sense of the person we have become.

We cannot divorce ourselves from the memories and experiences we have grown up with. Indeed, knowing, remembering and understanding them are vital for determining the changes that we might want to make for our future. Occasionally we don't recognise the unhelpful habits or behaviours that we haplessly imitate from our forebears. We need to understand, for example, the values our parents espoused since they probably guided their behaviour, which influenced how we behave and what we believe.

Indeed, we cannot overestimate how our own childhood is brought to bear in our experience as parents, in ways that we often don't realise until we face similar situations with our own children.

Understanding the parenting culture in which we were raised, how it affected us, and how we can make informed parenting choices that are not swayed by any remaining negative emotional consequences, provides us with some of the most powerful tools we will need in effective parenting.

If we know that elements of how we were reared had a negative impact on us, we may be eager to avoid replicating them in the lives and upbringing of our children. But unless we take time to question those values we will, unwittingly, live them out in our daily interactions. When it comes to our own family, we may require support, understanding and practical advice to avoid the pitfalls from our own past and to create the most wholesome environment for children to grow and develop. Gaining insight into the impact of our past experiences is the first step to creating our new future.

Understanding where we come from

We may have received harsh, rejecting or dismissive messages from our own parents, bosses or partners throughout our lives. We may not believe we are worthy or useful people. If we gain this insight, in adulthood, we must take on the challenge of overcoming it. Insight may come from feedback we get from friends, husbands, wives, partners, even our children. It may come from therapy, counselling or personal-development work that we do by ourselves or as part of our jobs. However we gain it, we must take responsibility for acting on it because we can only blame a bad childhood for so long! Eventually we need to take steps to change our limiting beliefs or behaviour.

Changing 'should' into 'could'

Perfectionism is a curse. Attending to detail and ensuring a high standard in what we do is good, but when that slips into absolutist inflexibility it is more likely to create stress or feelings of failure. These are just the kinds of dynamics that can arise for children if adults make too many demands of them without enough understanding.

While you were growing up, if you regularly felt you had failed to live up to your parents' expectations, you may carry that legacy forward unknowingly. If you hear yourself saying, 'I must …' or 'I should …' or 'I ought to …', the chances are that you set unreasonable expectations for yourself and probably always feel that you come up short or fail. Just as we will suggest with children, the aim is to do as much, or as best, as you can, rather than having some absolute standard that you 'must' reach.

Changing the word 'should' into the word 'could' is the quickest and most effective way to challenge our potential for unrealistic expectations of ourselves. When something 'could' or 'can' be done, it allows some freedom for not achieving it, unlike 'must'. By dint of being human we are imperfect. We can celebrate that imperfection rather than punish it.

Avoiding self-deprecation

Try to spot if you have a tendency to put yourself down, perhaps with phrases like 'I couldn't possibly …' or 'I was useless at Irish. Get your dad to help you with your homework …' Sometimes we grow into self-deprecation because pride in, and acknowledgement of, our achievements was seen as boasting. Sometimes self-deprecation is an extension of the rejection or dismissal we felt as a child.

We can challenge this kind of negative thinking and start to think positively instead. The first step is to notice when we think negatively and come up with a positive alternative. Perhaps try some positive self-talk or some self-affirmation like 'I am useful' or 'I deserve respect' or 'I can do many things'. When we repeat this type of phrase to ourselves daily, we may begin to believe it!

Accepting positive feedback

Many of us find it hard to accept compliments. We may often reject the positive feedback we receive from others. Notice if you hear yourself saying, 'It was nothing …' or 'I only did a tiny bit …' or 'Never mind that, did you see when I missed …'

We may often focus on the negative aspects of our performance and minimise the positive. This is another way of thinking that we can challenge. By being more mindful (and fair) we can start to listen to positive feedback and take note of it. If we have a predominantly negative outlook on life it can help us either to write down the good things people say about us and what we do, or to start noticing the good things ourselves and recording them. At the very least we will become more balanced when we have a long list of good stuff to offset the bad!

The importance of minding ourselves first

Over the years we may have slipped into unhealthy habits that put pressure on our bodies or add to psychological stress. If, based on our childhood experiences, we don't feel good about ourselves, it can be hard to bother minding ourselves.

However, looking after ourselves physically is also a way of looking positively towards the future. Be wary if you find you are constantly rushing; that you have little family time; that you have to do everything perfectly; that you suffer from sleeplessness and are overtired; that you rarely say, 'No,' to the demands made of you; that you're fretful; that you're under- or over-eating or that you become dependent upon alcohol or drugs. These are all signs that you're not minding yourself, and it is likely that you're not minding yourself because you don't feel worthy of being minded.

In your heart, you need to accept that you are worth caring for. You can show caring towards yourself by slowing down your lifestyle, eating healthily, taking regular exercise, socialising with friends, taking time for leisure, treating yourself, and by acting in a calm and relaxed way. In other words, allow yourself the qualities in life that you would wish for your children.

Living out core values in everyday life

So many of the problems we can identify in our lives today have their root in childhood. This is because, typically, our patterns of behaviour and ways of interacting with others were first learned when we were children. The values that we took from our families while we were growing up are the values that we, most likely, will bring to the family that we create. Values are, in essence, the ideas and beliefs we hold dear. They are the things that really matter to us; the things we feel should be held in high regard. In many ways our identities are an expression of the values we consider important.

For example, someone who values health will probably define themselves by the kinds of food they eat or the inclusion of regular exercise in their lives. Someone who values honesty will be seen to be truthful, and therefore reliable, based on their reactions to, and explanations of, various events in their daily lives. Someone who values responsibility will show themselves to follow through dependably on the tasks they take on or the commitments they make.

The core values that allow families to thrive

Imagine that in your family each child is empowered but not overpowering. They respect you and your authority but feel able to question and challenge the decisions that affect them. They are generous, thoughtful and kind to each other, to you and the wider community in which they live. They have goals and are self-motivated to achieve them. They are reliable and follow through on what they are asked or have volunteered to do.

I believe there are six values which, when we successfully live them out, create strong, thriving families:

1. Honesty
2. Trust
3. Respect
4. Kindness
5. Thoughtfulness
6. Responsibility

Prioritising our values

Most of us have more than one value that we hold dear. In fact, we can believe in many values, and those values tend to be held in a hierarchy. So, for example, if you value wealth and you also value honesty, when your tax return is due you will have to decide which value is predominant. If it is wealth, you may try to shelter or under-declare some income. If honesty is more important, you will declare all of your income even if it leaves you poorer.

Living our values in practice

Behaviour is the only accurate indicator of people's values. Values themselves are, in many ways, intangible and hidden. Many people will try to articulate their values in words, but it is only when we allow our values to prioritise or influence our behaviour that they become apparent to us and others. It's not enough to talk the talk, we must walk the walk too.

This is why, for example, children can feel confused by parents who demand respect by shouting at or hitting them. Neither shouting nor hitting is respectful behaviour so a child can feel a real conflict between their experience of disrespect from a parent and the insistence that they be respectful in their own behaviour towards that parent.

You and I are heavily influenced by what we saw, experienced and lived with in our families. Your parents may never have expressed their values to you in words, although it is quite likely that they did at some stage. What is more important, clearly, is what they showed you in their actions. In an ideal world their actions will have fitted with the values they espoused. How our parents actually lived their lives will be the truer indicator of the values they held. Those lived values will also be the stronger influence on our subsequent behaviour and attitudes. It is often only when we spot the difference between our parents' stated values and those they acted out that we may be spurred on to adopt and live a different set of values in our own and our families' lives.

Actions speak louder than words

I like to demonstrate the principle that actions speak louder than words in my public talks. I ask the audience to make an 'okay' symbol by touching the tip of their thumb to their index finger to make an o shape while spreading the other fingers of that hand. I demonstrate how to do this. Then I ask the audience to lift their right arms and wave the hand, still making the 'okay' symbol, from side to side. Again, I demonstrate this. I tell the audience to place that hand on their nose. For the first time I demonstrate something different. While telling them to put their hand on their nose, I am simultaneously placing mine on my cheek. The majority of the audience will ignore my verbal request, even if I repeat it, and copy what I do by placing their hand on their cheek.

Embracing our core values

Wherever we have picked up our values, from family, friends or even the wider society, the feedback we get from the world about how we live our lives may threaten or challenge some of those beliefs. Sometimes this will happen positively: for example, losing a friend as a result of lying to them may lead us to adopt honesty as a core value. Sometimes it is negative: having been an honest tax payer who lives among wide-scale tax fraud we may decide that if you can't beat them, you may as well join them, ditching honesty as a core value.

But if we have an awareness of the values we believe in, we can actively change or modify them. We don't have to be restricted by inherited values that we believe may be bad or limiting or may block us from thriving. If we want a thriving family, we need to adopt the values that will promote connectedness, good communication, nurturing, warmth and moral fortitude. We need values that allow us to be firm and kind. Honesty, trust, respect,

Even when I explain the principle before the demonstration, that we copy each other's actions and that our actions will override anything we might say, people still can't avoid copying my action. My words are in direct contradiction of my behaviour but my behaviour is always a more powerful influence on what people do. When there is discord between what a person is saying and doing, we decide that their behaviour is the better, or more accurate, indicator of what we should do.

Within families we find lots of discord between words and behaviour. For example, we can find ourselves shouting at our children to 'BE QUIET!' A child is more likely to copy the shout than obey the command. We tell our teenagers not to drink alcohol, yet we do so. We tell them to be responsible in their drinking, yet can be truly irresponsible ourselves.

kindness, thoughtfulness and responsibility will, I believe, create exactly that kind of thriving family. The essence of each value is outlined below.

1. Honesty

Honesty encompasses truthfulness, fairness, sincerity and integrity. It provides a foundation for many of the other important values that enable us to thrive. It is centrally important in trust, responsibility and respect. There is no doubt that when someone is honest with you, you know where you stand with him or her, and can relate more confidently and more successfully to them.

Truthfulness is a value we can struggle to engender in children. Children will often lie to avoid getting into trouble or getting others into trouble, to protect us from hurt or upset, or because they don't want to see or feel our reaction to their behaviour as it may cause embarrassment or shame. Of course, many adults lie for exactly the same reasons. In all cases the ultimate goal is to avoid the consequences of some action. Dishonesty, in this sense, reflects a real but understandable immaturity and lack of responsibility.

Sometimes the dishonest actions of our children can annoy, embarrass or shame us. We typically get angry with our children, forgetting that they are not ready to be fully aware of and responsible for their actions. We may, in fact, be misguided if we expect our pre-adolescent children to have evolved a moral sense of right and wrong because true conscience matures in adolescence.

Before this, children will usually do or avoid things on the basis of behavioural consequences for their previous actions, or on the basis of copying behaviour they witness around them. Lying and dishonesty fall into the same category of behaviour that children will engage in, or avoid, depending on how we parents typically respond to them and what we, as adults, present as a role model.

Consequently we need to be honest, sincere, fair and truthful in our dealings with our children, and we need to encourage them to tell the truth. In this way, the honesty they may display in childhood will be internalised so that by the time they reach adolescence they believe it is morally right to be honest.

Praising honesty over punishing dishonesty

Parents can unwittingly create the circumstances in which children will lie. If the climate in a house is one of punishment for wrongdoing, you are likely to be told more lies as an avoidance measure. Children can't help getting things wrong, and if they are fearful of the consequences of making mistakes, their first instinct will be to lie to avoid the punishment. Indeed, punishment may not reduce misbehaviour, but it will lead to under-reporting and evasion in the aftermath of such. The aim is to encourage children to want to tell the truth because they know they will be praised for their honesty, and that telling the truth will lead to lesser consequences.

Similarly, we can sometimes be keen to catch children out in the lies they tell us. We can use interrogatory questions to quiz them (often knowing the truth anyway), waiting for them to trip themselves up.

Sometimes we are simply encouraging them to talk enough that we can spot the lie and punish them for it. This, too, teaches children to be evasive and canny, rather than promoting honesty.

Role-modelling honesty includes acknowledging our mistakes and apologising to children as necessary. We frequently get it wrong, either in identifying the source of misbehaviour, choosing a fair and reasonable consequence, or misunderstanding or misinterpreting something a child says or does. However, many parents may feel afraid of diminishing their power by admitting to getting it wrong. In fact, saying that we made a mistake shows the honesty that underpins responsibility: a willingness to take ownership of what we say and do. It can only increase our stature and improve our relationship with our child.

We need to be sincere with our children. Sincerity can best be seen in saying what we mean and meaning what we say. There are times, usually in the heat of the moment, when we say things to children that we don't really intend. We might make a mean comment, or be dismissive of them, even though we hadn't intended to. We have a responsibility to think before we speak so that, as much as possible, we say only what we really mean.

Sometimes we make threats or promises to children that we have no intention (or ability) to follow through on. I've heard parents threaten to call the police and ask them to take children into care for their misbehaviour. I've heard parents threaten to ground a child for a month, even though they will probably have forgotten the threat after the first week. Equally, parents will fail to fulfil the promises they make. This could be about a small thing, like promising to read a story later, then forgetting. More significantly, a separated parent promises to visit their child, then fails to turn up. If children are to trust us and be disciplined by us, they must be able to believe what we tell them.

A final area in which we need to be honest with our children is in our expression of our feelings. Part of a child's emotional growth and development is their ability to recognise their own feelings and those of others. To achieve this they need to be able to make the connection between their feelings and their behaviour. It is important for them to see other people make these connections. We can unintentionally mask our true feelings in dealing with our children, which may confuse them as they try to make sense of different emotions.

For example, you may be taking your toddler to the park. If he lets go of your hand on the way and darts for the road, your understandable fright may lead you to grab his arm and respond angrily with words such as, 'Don't dare run out in the road – you could be killed!' In fact, the truer feeling we experience is more our own terror at the thought of him getting run over. A more honest statement to him would be, 'Don't let go of my hand. I'm terrified that a car will knock you over if you run out in the road.'

Talking honestly about our own feelings to children is a great way to boost their emotional development. Finding congruence, or a good fit, between how we feel and the experiences we have, and being able to demonstrate this to our children, shows them the path to emotional health and wellbeing.

2. Trust

Trust is a cornerstone of successful relationships. Families are an interconnected series of relationships and so, consequently, trust within families is vital. Many of the simple daily tasks we carry out rely on the commitment of other people to fulfil their side of a bargain. For example, we bring our child to the crèche and place complete trust in the staff to care for him or her.

All social contracts are based on trust. Depending on the situation, however, we may choose to write down the terms of an agreement we make with someone else. But a written contract shows recognition that we can't trust everybody. What we are effectively saying to the other person is, 'I don't fully trust you to deliver on what we have agreed so I am writing it all down. If you don't do what you say you are going to do, someone else [a court, for example] will punish you for breaking our agreement.' Somewhere in the development of society we have come to understand that while we need to be able to trust other people to get through the business of the day, not everyone will be worthy of that trust. Not everyone is honest.

As with written contracts, we often suggest there will be consequences for the other person if they prove to be untrustworthy, even in verbal agreements. Families are no different in this regard. So much of the trust that we place in each other, within our families, is also conditional. For example, with a thirteen- or fourteen-year-old, we may say, 'I trust you to come straight out from the disco at 11 p.m. and I will be waiting to collect you. If you don't turn up on time, I will have to reconsider letting you go to another disco in the future.'

The stated desire to trust your child is there. They have two potential motivators in action to help them stick by the agreement: first, they may believe it is a good thing and so have internal motivation to want to be trustworthy; second, they may just want to avoid the consequence of being late.

I believe that a person's motivation to be trustworthy is less important than his or her behaviour, because trust is built on the basis of behavioural evidence. So, if someone says they are going to do something and follows through, we can begin to believe that they are reliable and trustworthy. The more times they show this reliability and consistency, the more we will feel they can be trusted and relied upon.

How trust is formed

eBay, the online auction and marketplace, places huge emphasis on buyer and seller ratings as a means of trying to display the participants' relative trustworthiness. After each transaction you are encouraged to rate the other person about the extent to which you each fulfilled your side of the bargain.

A seller will rate the buyer on whether payment came through in full and on time, and a buyer will rate the seller on whether the goods arrived in a timely fashion and as advertised. The site cannot function unless its users have confidence that the items they are selling or buying will be paid for or delivered as described.

Even the ratings system is not enough to give every user the confidence that the deal they strike online will be honoured. PayPal, the online payments portal, has grown out of the need for a third-party, independent entity that can straddle the divide between buyer and seller, giving confidence to each that they have some level of protection if the deal goes bad.

It is the behavioural nature of how trust is demonstrated that makes it so hard to evaluate and depend on in social interactions and contracts. There is no yardstick we can use to determine someone's trustworthiness. Equally, we can't prove to anyone that we are trustworthy. All we will ever have is whatever evidence we can produce of our previous activity and how trustworthy it can be deemed to have been.

On the flip side, if someone promises something and fails to deliver it, we feel disappointed, hurt, perhaps even betrayed, and are less likely to trust them again because they have let us down. Depending on the situation, one experience of let-down can negate months or even years of trust. This is a dilemma we face with children. We know we need to trust them for them to grow and thrive, but actually they will often betray that trust simply because they make mistakes. We have to bite the bullet each time and extend our trust again (even if we fear they'll make a mess of it again!).

If you grew up with a core distrust in your parents because they let you down throughout your childhood and adolescence, you may find it difficult to make the initial leap of faith to trust anyone, let alone your children. If you saw in your parents' relationship the evidence that they couldn't and didn't trust each other, you will have learned to be wary of others' reliability.

Equally, if your faith in the trustworthiness of others has been rocked by small or large betrayals, you may be more focused, and even fixated, on the varying levels of trustworthiness that your family shows. Your hyper-vigilance or wariness may block the development of trust in your family. You may believe that 'you can't trust anybody in life'.

In fact, you can trust everybody in life; what you can't guarantee is that everyone will uphold the trust you place in them. So, rather than approaching the world in a distrustful way, we can approach it trustingly. What we then learn is that there are some people we can continue to trust and some we can't. Even though there are no guarantees, developing a sense of trust in the world is a positive thing.

3. Respect

When we think about respect we usually consider two aspects: respect as a form of admiration or recognition, and respect as a form of deference or obeisance. Respect is about acknowledging the value in other people. When we feel respected by someone, it helps reinforce our self-esteem. We feel valued because we are either likeable or have some appealing ability or abilities.

Conversely, if we feel disrespected by someone, we may assume there is something wrong with us. We may feel undervalued or that we possess some personality flaw that makes us unattractive or unlikeable. Contempt is the opposite of respect and reflects the complete absence of care that some people will show to others.

Respect and love are intricately bound together. We can respect someone else without loving them, but we cannot love them without respecting them. Although love is not all that your children need, they cannot thrive without love and respect.

The importance of unconditional love

True love is the acceptance of another person without any strings attached. We all come with our abilities and faults, our failings and successes. Loving our children means accepting their good and bad days equally. It means accepting that they are different from us, and allowing their personality to grow, develop and be celebrated. When a child feels loved, it gives them the courage and confidence to be an individual while feeling intimately connected to other people. To know that we are loved nourishes the very centre of our being and sends a very strong message that we are valued and respected by someone else.

Ironically, when you ask most parents what it means for their children to respect them, they will consider the extent to which their children comply with their requests or demands. When children are not compliant, they are often considered disrespectful. In fact non-compliance may also be the result of tiredness, anger, a sense of injustice, laziness or misunderstanding of what was requested.

We need to be careful, therefore, not to associate respect only with compliance. Indeed, sometimes children will comply with demands out of fear, not respect. So, using compliance as a measure of respect is flawed.

Regularly, in my clinical practice, parents complain to me of their children's disrespect. They complain that their children ignore them or speak dismissively to them. They complain that their children are deliberately oppositional. They complain that their children act wilfully and boldly as if to prove that they have more power than the parent.

Much as I mentioned earlier, I often find that a pattern of disrespect first became apparent in the parent's treatment of their child. I may discover that such parents shout frequently at their children, or apply harsh punishments, or disregard their child's opinion and perspective. Rarely is this done intentionally, yet if parents exert (or try to exert) a lot of power with no moderating sense of understanding or kindness it can often result in disrespectful children who may simply be copying the behaviour of their parents.

Similar dynamics will be seen in other areas where people in positions of power feel disrespected. Some sports coaches who lose the respect of their players will have wielded a lot of authority and made heavy demands of the players without being responsive to them and their needs. Some teachers who complain of disrespect among students will, similarly, have been highly authoritarian with no tempering consideration of the youngsters' perspective.

When children grow up in an atmosphere of disrespect, they may transfer their disrespect to any authority figure. So, there are times when, no matter what we do in a position of authority, we will be faced with disrespect from some people who may just have grown to be contemptuous. When such children gain a position of power, their contempt for others can lead to bullying in child- and adulthood. For example, a child who learns that they can frighten other children by being threatening, and thereby get their own way, may continue to threaten because they don't care how the other children are feeling and because they enjoy the comparative security that the feeling of power engenders.

When I meet teenagers in my clinical practice their most common complaint is that nobody listens to them. This is often ironic since their parents will equally complain that their teenagers no longer talk to them. In fact, the experience of those teenagers is that they are listened to but not heard: they feel their opinions and beliefs are neither valued nor respected. The parents are not showing that they understand or recognise the value in their youngster in the way he or she is seeking.

So, if we want our families to thrive, we must show our children that we respect them. We can do this by being firm (to show them we care about their safety and wellbeing) but, crucially, by also showing understanding and being responsive to them. We must show that we have regard for and are considerate of them. The respect that we show will be returned and our children will grow up to be respectful of other people, whether they are in authority or not.

4. Kindness

My mother always told me, 'A little bit of kindness goes a long way.' It was only when I had grown up that I began to work out for myself what kindness went a long way towards: strong relationships. We know intuitively when someone is being kind to us in the small things they might do for us that seem above and beyond the call of duty; they show caring and consideration.

Often we may feel we don't deserve the kindnesses shown to us, although we invariably feel nurtured, loved and cared about when we do experience kindness from others. That, in turn, will lead us to feel warmly and considerately towards whoever was kind to us so a connection is either established or strengthened. Being kind to children, when they least expect it, reinforces the positive elements of your relationship with them. Being kind regularly gives them a solid base from which they can grow and thrive.

Having kindness at the heart of our family experience will nurture a sense of altruism (selflessness and concern for the needs of others). This concept, that we must align our own fortunes with those of others, is at the heart of community. Families are communities in their own right but they are also the building blocks for wider communities in society. We are social beings and we are more inclined to thrive when we work with others rather than against them.

Learning to share depends on trust and kindness. Most people learn to share on the basis that 'what goes around comes around'. If I am generous with the world, the world will be generous with me.

Good for the giver

Researchers have coined the term a 'helper's high' to describe the natural and profound sense of wellbeing and optimism that comes from being kind to others. In the US they have found that states with higher rates of volunteerism have lower rates of heart disease. Another study, published in the *Journal of Health Psychology*, followed about six hundred older adults. After adjusting for differences in socioeconomic status, prior health status, smoking, social support and physical activity, volunteerism decreased death rates by more than 44 per cent. So, being kind to others doesn't just benefit the receiver: it also nourishes the giver, emotionally and physically.

Having kindness ingrained as a value will make our family life feel warm and connected. Great family experiences are rooted in connectedness, when we feel goodwill and care for those who are around us. Sometimes I wrap up the ideas of kindness and warmth in the term 'nurturing'. Nurturing, for me, brings up feelings of being minded, cared about, swaddled, protected and safe.

How we nurture our children says a lot about how we value kindness. It doesn't cost much to be kind, yet in the flurry of daily life it's easy to lose our warmth towards our children. Annoyance with how a day is going can spill over so that our children bear the brunt of our frustration. Thinking kindly of our children doesn't mean having to be nice to them no matter what, or having to give in to them all the time. Thinking kindly of them might, however, lead to a less sharp tone, less criticism, less dismissal and more acceptance of their natural imperfections. Sometimes kindness might lead to a hug when we, or they, least expect it and most need it.

Selflessness is required of parents. We often put ourselves out for our children and for each other. We often have to go the extra mile to keep our families going, never mind thriving, and it is very hard to keep giving unless we receive something in return. Indeed, as parents, the amount of work we do often goes unrecognised and unacknowledged.

Sometimes generosity of spirit will get us through. For many of us, the satisfaction of seeing our children thrive, enjoy themselves, grow, develop and be happy is enough reinforcement of our giving and generosity. However, we may at times have felt it hasn't been enough to sustain the effort we put in. There are times when we need our efforts to be recognised.

If we don't get any kind of positive reinforcement for the selflessness we show, it is easy to feel taken for granted, which can lead to growing bitterness. It is almost impossible for kindness to thrive in a culture of bitterness. Parents will start to do the minimum required, children will feel the tension, resentment and anger, and they will grow selfish and demanding rather than kind and generous. Alternatively, embittered parents may continue to do the lion's share of the work but will try to make their children, and others, feel guilty about their non-contribution. Such parents may end up shaming their children into contributing even though this will likely leave the children feeling resentful and unwilling, far from the generosity that the parent hopes for.

To avoid bitterness setting in we have to be clear with ourselves, and our families, about the kind of feedback and acknowledgement we want for our efforts. We start early with children, encouraging them to say, 'Ta,' when, as babies and toddlers, they are given something. Some of this is about politeness, but some of it is about teaching children that generosity, kindness and giving should not be taken for granted.

5. Thoughtfulness

Thoughtfulness involves showing consideration for other people. Being thoughtful requires us to put ourselves in someone else's place and see the world from their perspective. In particular we can be conscious of another's feelings and react compassionately towards them. Thoughtfulness is the precursor to kindness and responsiveness in dealing with our children. Thoughtfulness will balance our firmness and expectations of them.

For example, a thoughtful father trying to get his reluctant three-year-old into the car may say something like, 'You've been having great fun and it's hard when play has to stop and we have to go home. But it's time to get into the car, even if you don't want to.' That statement acknowledges what the child is likely to be feeling: understandable frustration and disappointment at having to go home. The father still holds the limit and gets his son into the car but he is understanding and considerate of the upset it might cause.

A similar father who is under pressure and has neither the time nor the inclination to be thoughtful may say, 'Okay, time to go. Get into the car. If you don't get in by yourself then I'll put you in!' Again, there is no doubt that the dad will get his son into the car, but by doing so in an authoritarian way, which fails to acknowledge the child's feelings, it is much more likely to result in his son having a full-blown tantrum!

As mentioned, one aspect of being thoughtful is the ability to recognise how someone else is feeling. This is known as empathy. Empathy is one of the most important skills that thriving families develop and use. When parents can empathise with their children, we find that so much more of their behaviour becomes explicable, even if it remains unacceptable.

A child who is jealous of their little sister may hit her with a toy. Being able to empathise with the older child's jealousy allows us to understand why he or she may have been aggressive. It doesn't make it okay that they hit their little sister but it does mean that we can think further about a good way to respond to the hitting.

One option is to punish the older child, which will probably lead to further resentment and dislike of their sibling. Another is to help him or her to understand their own jealousy so that they are not reacting to it passively. A clear, acknowledging statement can be a much more productive way of dealing with such a situation: 'I think you feel jealous of all the attention your sister gets and you may get quite angry about that. However, even if you feel cross and jealous you may not hit her. If you feel cross with your sister, come and tell me and I'll help.'

Thoughtfulness requires that we think! So, taking a step back from a situation means that we don't react in the heat of the moment. By pausing, perhaps taking some time out and away from the incident, we can consider the different perspectives, including how our children are feeling, and we may spot how those feelings may be influencing their behaviour. When we have paused to calm ourselves from our own feelings of, for example, indignation or anger, we can start to see the bigger picture. Often when we can see the world from our children's perspective, too, we may choose to moderate or change our own responses to their behaviour.

The difference between empathy and sympathy

Empathy requires us to see the world from someone else's perspective so that we can imagine or guess how they might feel. It doesn't require us to share that feeling with them. For instance, I can empathise with a child whose father has died; even though I haven't experienced my own father's death I can make an educated guess at what that child might feel although I don't feel any of the same terrible loss, hurt or distress. Sympathy is what we experience when we share the same feeling as someone else. I can sympathise with my brother about our granny dying because we share the experience of being her grandsons and probably have quite similar feelings of missing her. When children feel distressed, upset, hurt, angry or experience any other emotion, it is enough for us to empathise with them. They don't need us to have the same feelings. They just want us to be thoughtful enough to understand how they feel.

Thoughtfulness also promotes mindfulness. Mindfulness is attending to what is happening in the present moment in contrast with more habitual states of mind in which we are often preoccupied with memories, fantasies, worries or planning. Mindfulness has been shown to reduce mental-health difficulties, such as depression and anxiety, by helping us tune into our feelings and stopping us dwelling on the past or worrying about the future. Then we get more out of the day-to-day.

More than many other values, a thoughtful, heedful and careful approach to life will build strong connected relationships within our family. The more connected we are, the more we can promote other values, like respect, responsibility and trust.

6. Responsibility

If we are responsible for something, we are liable to be called on to answer for our behaviour: we may be praised or punished for what we do because we accept that we chose to behave in a particular way. Being responsible can also mean being reliable and trustworthy. In this sense it refers to dependability and following through, or completing, our obligations.

Sometimes we use these different meanings interchangeably and at others we intend to mean just one or the other. When we refer to a 'responsible adult' (perhaps leading a group of schoolchildren on a tour), both meanings apply: that adult is a reliable individual whom we trust to take care of the children and return them safely;

he or she may also be in charge and therefore liable for sanction if anything goes wrong.

There are times when I would rather not have to take the consequences for things I have done. I have clear recollections from my childhood of trying to evade responsibility for my actions. Children and teenagers can't be fully responsible in the way adults are expected to be. Indeed, irresponsibility is a natural part of childhood, and the ability and willingness to take full responsibility is a mark of true adulthood.

Children naturally avoid responsibility

Once, when I was twelve or thirteen, I took some money from the kitchen at home. When my parents noticed it was missing they asked my brother and me about it. I denied any knowledge. I remember my dad warning us that the punishment for taking the money would be less if the culprit owned up. After a few agonising hours of self-recrimination, fear and guilt, I told my parents that I'd taken the money. I don't recall any particularly harsh punishment, but I do remember my dad commenting that not owning up to the stealing was as bad as the stealing itself. He recognised that I had made a mistake in taking the money but he also understood that trying to avoid the consequences was an equally natural mistake.

Children need adults around them to set the boundaries and guide their behaviour. If a five-year-old child is given a bag of sweets, we may expect him or her to eat the lot in one sitting so we take away the bag and decide how many sweets they can have at a time so that they enjoy the treat without feeling sick. We do this because working out the consequences of an action requires foresight that children and teenagers may not have. Developing the ability to plan ahead and predict consequences relies upon the frontal lobes of the brain (the bit behind our foreheads). The frontal cortex is the last part of the brain to mature: we are in our early twenties before it reaches full maturity.

Teenagers and children make irresponsible mistakes because they can't or don't see beyond their immediate behaviour so cannot be held liable for it. This is why courts and the legal system don't prosecute or punish juveniles according to the same standards as adults. Children have diminished responsibility because they may not be mature enough to grasp the full consequences of their actions.

We need to teach children about consequences, rather than just punish them for their mistakes. Homes in which punishment for 'wrongdoing' is frequent and significant produce conformist children who grow up, in the main, to be quite conformist adults. These children, and the adults they become, conform simply because they are afraid of the consequences of not doing so. These adults retain a comparatively immature sense of responsibility. For example, a highly conformist person is more likely to park their car legally to avoid being clamped rather than to reduce the traffic disruption that may be caused if it is parked illegally and in the way of other traffic.

We need to find ways to encourage our children to accept liability for their actions. We want them to grow into their responsibility so, even though they will regularly make mistakes along the way, we must increasingly give them more choices and more opportunities to take responsibility. When they get things wrong, our aim is to show them where and why things went wrong so that they can learn to do better or differently the next time.

We can also demonstrate being responsible, in the sense of being reliable and owning up to our own behaviour, so that they learn from us. If we behave responsibly, our children are more likely to be responsible too. We want our children eventually to 'stand up and be counted' but to achieve this we have to do the same along the way.

Living our values in daily life

It is a challenge to uphold these six values every day. We must believe in them and act in accordance with them. Family life is a complex system of intertwined relationships that occur in a wide range of supportive and/or challenging environments. None of us is perfect, and there are days when we patently make mistakes in rearing our children and our family doesn't thrive. However, if our intentions are sound, we stand a better chance of creating the atmosphere in which it can.

There are times when I don't always live by the values I aspire to, but I mean well and I try hard. I do the best I can. I believe that this will be good enough for my family to thrive. If your heart is in the right place, this book will show you how to create a happy, strong and nurturing home that will be good enough for your family to thrive.

02
THRIVING FROM THE START OF FAMILY LIFE

'How come nobody told us?'
Adjusting to parenthood

Becoming a parent for the first time is a complete whirlwind. It can be emotionally, psychologically and physically overwhelming. For the first time we are directly, personally and explicitly responsible for the life of another. This is a big deal. On top of that, we're trying to come to terms with our new role in life, our sleep is disrupted, we're tuned to almost every breath our baby takes, and there is probably a flurry of well-wishers and supportive helpers to attend to. It's no wonder we feel frazzled.

The early weeks and months of family life pass in a blur of late nights, early mornings, nappies, cleaning, washing, feeding, burping and pacing the floor with a disgruntled tot in our arms. Some days we don't even make it out of our pyjamas. In the past a pyjama day may have signalled downtime and relaxation. Now it is testament to how our lives have been taken over by another.

Somewhere within this potential chaos and the fog of exhaustion we are meant to know exactly what to do at every hour and in every situation to meet the needs of our babies and to sow the seeds of a successful family life. It is hard to conceive of the kind of family we want to create, and how we can thrive, when we can barely think at all.

Merging instinct with intention

Coping with a brand-new arrival is as much to do with instinct as with planning or intention. We have many intuitive and unconscious responses to our babies that we can't explain, other than that it seemed the right thing to do in that moment. There will be elements of our instinctive responses that we will question and perhaps seek advice about, but mostly we'll just get on with it. Thinking about family, values and traditions, hopes and expectations, legacy and baggage that we may carry will come later. In fact, real thinking about any of these things may happen only when intuition seems to fail us.

When things seem to 'work' in a family, we rarely question what we do or why we do it. It is often only when things seem to stop working that we wonder why and, more importantly, what can we do about it. These are the times when we make explicit, if only to ourselves, our core beliefs about what makes a family function well, what we hope for and intend with our family.

In an ideal world, we will have time with our partners to discuss all of this, even at the start of family life. Perhaps we had the foresight to do it before our babies were born. Discussing our beliefs about family will allow us to find common ground in how we might approach different situations. It will allow us to discover what beliefs we share and where our views diverge.

'A good start' is half the work

It's easy to feel overwhelmed at the beginning of family life. So many of the situations we find ourselves in are new and we may have little idea of how to negotiate them successfully. But what we do at the start will often determine how we continue. For example, if one partner takes on the main burden of parenting and housework, they may end up permanently assigned to those roles. Or, if your gut response to your baby's cries is to get angry with him or her for being unreasonable, you may find that your resentment at the responsibility they have brought with them will increase throughout their childhood.

There is an old Irish saying 'Tús maith, leath na hoibre', meaning 'A good start is half the work.' This is as true in determining the kind of family experience we will create for our children as it is in many other areas. Pure natural instinct, our intuitive sense of what to do, will get us along some of the road to where we might want to go, but our instinct is not only based on what nature intends: it is also significantly shaped by our own family upbringing and how our parents created their family.

Learning to recognise our unconscious responses

Some of our unconscious responses to our babies and children will be the result of what we have learned to do. Even if our parents don't turn up on our doorstep with good wishes and lots of advice, they will be influencing indirectly our interactions with our baby. If they do turn up to visit, their well-meaning interventions, advice and at times explicit direction may increase our feelings of stress. Our parents have a lot of lived experience when it comes to raising a family. In theory they should know how to do it well. But our experiences of being part of their family will also sway how much we want to let them be part of our new family.

Perhaps you had a relatively happy upbringing and your parents were good enough. Now you may welcome their support, understanding and advice with open arms. But if you feel they failed you at critical times in your life, you may not want them to influence your son or daughter in the same, or similar, negative ways. Indeed, it may seem perfectly obvious that if you felt your parents didn't do a good job with you, you wouldn't want them to be involved in your child's life. In reality, however, we can often be blind to the mistakes of the past, either unknowingly or deliberately. Many of us yearn to forgive the hurts we experienced in the hope that things will be better or different in the future.

Feeling secure and confident

Our own circumstances at the time of the birth are also important factors in how we settle into our newly extended family. Our sense of stability is crucially important. If we feel we have solid ground under our feet, it can free us to find our way confidently through some of the parenting dilemmas we will face. Single, married, gay, straight, entering a new family situation with or without step-children: these issues are less important than feeling secure about our place in the world.

However, feeling isolated or worried because a relationship feels weakened or has broken down during the pregnancy may unsettle anyone in the early stages of family life. Similarly, major changes, such as moving house, or adversities, such as bereavement or job loss, may result in increased levels of anxiety and stress so that a family's focus may be simply on surviving more than thriving. Even in the midst of turmoil, however, a strong sense of self and a clear sense of direction will be of invaluable help to us to continue striving to make our family life the best it can be.

Achieving a strong sense of self means determining the values we believe in. We need to think about what is good for us and our family, so that we can be proactive in making decisions rather than simply reactive. Before we had children, we may have described ourselves in terms of our occupation. Now that we are parents too, or instead, we need to consider what kind of parents we want to be.

Learning to accept help

It can be tempting, at times, to become insular in caring for our babies. Have you ever found yourself thinking things like 'Only I can get her to sleep', or 'She'll only feed well for me', or 'Give him back to me; only I can settle him'? Sometimes we lack trust in the capability of others to look after our baby, as much as we worry at other times about our own.

There is a lovely old African saying that translates roughly as 'It takes a village to raise a child.' It suggests that communal support for families and communal influence on children and their upbringing are of real benefit in helping them to thrive. We are social beings, and most of the time when we work together we can achieve more than if we work alone. Trusting others is central to achieving this. Trust is a big deal. It requires a certain level of faith in humanity. For a society to function, we must trust others in small and big ways.

Naturally, how much we can trust other people may have been influenced by our experiences within our own families growing up. The more reliable our parents were when we were children and teenagers, the more we are likely to have grown up as trustworthy and trusting adults ourselves. As babies, the ideal start was to have experienced the world as a safe, predictable and reliable place. Allowing babies to develop trust early in their lives will provide them with solid bedrock upon which they can move forward and thrive. How do we achieve this?

Building secure attachments and developing trust

When we trust other people at a core level we feel more secure. But when and where is that security, or insecurity, first experienced? Our earliest experiences of trust came at our birth and in the two or three years that followed. Those early years are critical to how we develop trust and security for it is then that attachment develops.

Attachment takes time

Attachment is a psychological process in which an infant connects itself emotionally and psychologically to an adult. To survive, an infant must have an adult to take care of it. In the early weeks after birth a baby will produce sounds, cry and make eye contact with any adult available. They will try to attract attention so that their needs are met. Naturally, for most babies the same person is there to respond.

From around two months, babies begin to discriminate and develop growing awareness of who primarily meets their needs. Typically this is their mother, although we often use the term 'primary care-giver' to acknowledge that they could also be a father, an extended family member or even another carer, such as a foster parent. At this stage an infant becomes more discerning about who looks after them and may only become settled, for example, when they are comforted by their primary care-giver. Between the ages of six months and two to three years, babies and toddlers come to rely upon this person not only for their physical but also their emotional needs, for comfort and security.

Reassuringly, this means that we have many opportunities throughout those first three years to be reliable and consistent enough for a secure attachment to develop. This developmental window is comparatively large so we can change and adjust what we do to increase our trustworthiness, and know that it can make a big difference to our babies or toddlers. This is because attachment is built up on the basis of a parent's continued responses to their baby's needs. Secure attachment means that a baby can rely upon its parents to meet its needs consistently and warmly. Because the parents' behaviour is reliable and predictable, their baby can learn to trust them.

How we learn to trust

Babies come to know how trustworthy a parent is by the dependable way in which he or she responds to their efforts to attract attention. The more often and more consistently a parent responds to their baby's needs (to be held, fed, cleaned, soothed and kept warm and comfortable), the more evidence the baby will have that their parent is trustworthy.

How well equipped that adult is to meet these needs consistently will determine how secure the child's attachment is. In essence a mother or father must show her- or himself to be trustworthy and dependable for the child to learn about trust. When children learn that they can trust their parents, by extension they learn to trust others too. With a secure attachment in place, a child will feel able to explore their world, safe in the knowledge that their parents can be trusted to intervene if need be.

Challenges to building secure attachment

Children can also feel insecure in their attachment to their parent. Research tells us that about four out of ten children's sense of trust is disrupted. Chronic neglect, untreated post-natal depression, other mental-health problems for parents, physical or sexual abuse within a family, chronic alcohol or other addictions can all mean that we can't or don't provide good enough care for our children. Most children who end up in the social care system will have experienced early challenges in their relationship formation.

But, thankfully, children are resilient, and in most cases if we make ourselves reliable and trustworthy and show this in how we care for and love them, our children will grow to trust us, feeling secure and loved. If their early experiences were neglectful, traumatic or chaotic, the process will be harder, but not impossible.

A case in point ...

Anna contacted me for an appointment about three weeks after her daughter was born. She was very worried that she hadn't bonded with her baby. She told me her daughter's birth had been traumatic, ending in a forceps delivery. She described vividly that it felt 'like she was being ripped out of me. I felt like I failed her by not being able to push properly.' She spoke of how mothers are supposed to feel 'this rush of love' towards their babies but that she didn't at the time, and hadn't since.

Anna felt obliged to care for her daughter rather than wanting to. She had read a lot in advance of the birth and was now worried that her and her baby's attachment wasn't good. Even though she felt she should be doing more, she admitted finding it hard to do all the things that her baby seemed to demand. Bravely, she even acknowledged that there were times when she almost wished her daughter hadn't been born because she really felt she couldn't do 'the whole mothering thing'.

Although we often use the terms bonding and attachment interchangeably, they actually refer to two different things. Attachment is the long process by which infants connect to, and come to trust, their primary care-giver. Bonding is the process by which a parent feels emotionally connected to their infant. Bonding typically happens in the minutes, hours and days after the birth to ensure that the adult sticks around to care for their helpless infant.

Although a mother is physiologically and psychologically primed to bond with her baby, I explained to Anna that it doesn't always work out like this, especially when the mother is coping with the aftermath of a traumatic birth, as in Anna's case. Anna may not have bonded with her baby, but there were good reasons for this. Her difficult birth experience had been a massive shock to her system, and probably numbed all of her feelings. I explained that this is a very natural strategy for dealing, in the short term, with overwhelmingly strong emotions. There was nothing for her to feel bad about or, necessarily, anything to block her from bonding, in time, with her daughter.

Since Anna had done a lot of reading around the subject, I reminded her that in the early weeks her daughter just needed someone to meet her needs in a timely and consistent manner. So, if Anna felt unable to carry out certain duties, it was fine to let her husband, her mother or any other capable adult take over. Indeed, Anna's motivation for responding to her daughter was less important than the fact that she did respond to her. Even if it was obligation, not desire, which led her to pick up her daughter, to feed or change her, that was good enough to help her daughter's attachment to develop securely.

I reassured Anna that, by crying, her daughter was simply telling her that she needed something. I explained that, like all parents, Anna must try to work out what this was (often a process of trial and error). As long as she was warm and responsive in meeting her baby's needs, that was good enough right then. I suggested to her that she rely more on the support of the other people around her so that she had a little time to mind herself. Unless our own needs are met it is almost impossible to meet someone else's. For Anna to mind her baby, she needed to feel minded. [to be continued]

Practical ways to build a secure attachment

Even if the early weeks and months of our babies' lives are a struggle, emotionally, physically and psychologically, for them and us, attachments can and do form securely. In fact, we have the first two or three years of their lives to establish that connection. There are practical things we can do to build secure relationships with our babies. The best ways of connecting to babies and, crucially, letting them connect to us are touching, holding, talking to and playing with them.

I have found that the practices listed below make a big difference to the amount of trust a baby can place in its care-giver, and consequently to the quality and security of the attachment they develop.

* **Make eye contact.** Babies will naturally seek to focus on the eyes of adults who care for them. Looking at your baby and locking your gaze with theirs is a powerful indicator that you are physically and emotionally present to mind them.

❈ **Smile and talk to your child.** Babies and toddlers who can't yet speak will babble away to the world. Responding to that babbling, by acknowledging it with a smile and dignifying it with a response, shows your child that they are noticed and reassures them that they can get your attention without having to cry.

❈ **Express warmth and touch.** Picking children up, giving babies a massage and stroking a toddler's back will express an element of nurturing to a baby or child. Children who feel nurtured feel more secure.

❈ **Be sensitive and responsive.** Babies who cry are trying to tell you that they need something from you. They are not persecuting you (although any parent will know that it can feel like that sometimes!) so the more gentle and calm we can be in responding to them the more they are soothed and the more they will grow to trust that others are there for them.

❈ **Get in tune with your child.** Most of us quickly learn the different cries our babies make, be it for hunger, tiredness or discomfort. Being in tune with what they are trying to tell us at the pre-verbal stage allows us to meet their needs more quickly and easily, and keeps them contented.

❈ **Follow your child's lead in play.** As your baby grows into a toddler, devoting time to playing together is a further opportunity to allow them to feel attended to. Try to let the play be on their terms, as this helps them to rely, yet again, on your ability to be responsive to them.

❈ **Read together.** Reading to your child is a nurturing activity that often leads to a wonderful feeling of warmth and safety for a child who is typically snuggled up beside or on you. Never mind the imaginative stimulation it provides; often its most powerful benefit is the closeness it brings.

When we do these things with our babies and children, they feel recognised, noticed and loved. That gives them confidence that we can be relied upon. Once they have this secure base in us, they can go and explore their world, trusting that we will still be there, if needed, to make everything better.

Thriving as a result of secure attachment

There is a real benefit to be gained by working hard on building attachments.

❀ Children who are secure in their attachments explore their environment with greater freedom and are able to learn with confidence.

❀ Children who are secure tend to be more popular with peers and exhibit more positive social interaction with other children.

❀ Children who are secure tend to be more emotionally stable and able to express and manage their feelings well as they get older.

❀ Children who are secure demonstrate greater ability to handle stress and help others handle it.

Post-natal depression and a struggle to thrive

Having a baby is supposed to be a wonderful experience, but it can also be completely overwhelming. We have some major readjustments to make in the aftermath, with the loss of our independence, an increased sense of responsibility, significantly reduced sleep and changes in our finances, along with trying to get our heads around our new roles as mother, father and no longer being simply a couple. Under these circumstances, it seems normal to feel emotionally vulnerable and sensitive; often, the time when we are most called upon to mind another is when we need to be minded ourselves.

More than the 'baby blues'

About half of all new mothers describe having the 'baby blues' after the birth of their child. This can involve feeling grumpy and irritable as well as tearful. Indeed, you may feel as if your emotions are constantly changing so you feel very unsettled. Often mothers feel they have no confidence in their ability to look after their baby. This often happens between three and five days after the birth and may coincide with hormonal changes, as the natural high often experienced after childbirth passes and the realities of a new routine come to the fore: being alone in charge of their baby after discharge from hospital, and the understandable exhaustion of those early days. With the reassurance and support of partners, friends and family, the baby blues usually pass in a week or so.

Post-natal depression (PND) is different. It affects between 10 and 15 per cent, or around one in eight, of all mothers. Fathers can also experience depression after the birth of a child. The symptoms of PND continue for weeks and months after the birth. The most common symptoms are:

* Low mood and feeling upset
* General anxiety (sometimes with panic attacks)
* Constant worry about the baby
* Feeling exhausted but unable to sleep
* Unable to look forward to anything.

Sometimes we miss the signs of PND because they may be masked by the chronic lack of sleep and exhaustion that most parents experience in the first few months as their baby's daily rhythm settles.

Factors that increase the risk of developing PND

❀ History of depression, mental-health issues or PND

❀ Difficult labour or traumatic delivery

❀ Few friends or family to help or support

❀ Being a one-parent family

❀ A sick, cross or hard-to-settle baby

❀ A child with a disability

❀ Death of your own parent during pregnancy

❀ Financial pressure

❀ Any other significant stressor on the family or parent.

A case in point, continued ...

After my initial session with Anna, in which I had tried to reassure her about her ability to build a secure attachment for her baby, I hadn't anticipated seeing her again. However, I later discovered that within the few months after the birth her sense of disconnection with her baby deepened and she developed post-natal depression. During this time she felt unable to contact me or reach out for help in any way. These were dark days for Anna.

Months later, when she finally came to see me, she said she had felt as if her whole world had been about to fall apart. She felt exhausted and overwhelmed by having this tiny person whom she felt was reliant on her alone. It was like being stuck in a downward spiral. Her daughter cried a lot (she had bad reflux), and the more she cried, the less Anna felt she coped.

Anna felt helpless to soothe her daughter, yet trapped by her obligation to care for her. She felt constantly overcome by anxiety, afraid to let her baby out of her sight, convinced she was the only one who could properly look after her, yet at the same time *dreading the long days alone with her. She grew apart from her husband, who didn't understand, she thought, and couldn't help anyway. She felt truly isolated. One day she recalled her anxiety turning to a burning rage. She was furious at what she saw as her own weakness and incompetence as a mother. She banged her head hard against the wall, feeling the pain but also realising she must do something. She went to her GP, who prescribed anti-depressants, and came back to me.*

We worked on and off over the next couple of years on practical things that Anna could do to continue to support her daughter's attachment, despite her own emotional struggles. We also looked at the trauma of the birth, Anna's sense that she was out of control and her subsequent exhausting attempts to over-control every situation and be all things to her daughter while resenting and barely coping with the effort involved.

We worked hard at allowing Anna to reconnect with her husband, and including and involving him in a meaningful way in their daughter's care. Anna allowed herself to accept his support and that of her extended family. She looked out beyond her role as mother and made sure to take regular walks for herself, then became a phone support for other mothers with PND.

In time her depression lifted, between the medication, the therapy and her own efforts to be active. Most importantly, though, Anna came to see that her daughter's attachment to her was secure. Despite the rocky start, she had shown her daughter that she was reliable and dependable enough to be trusted. Anna saw that post-natal depression, and the early struggle of parenting, did not destroy her daughter or herself. A parent–child relationship is resilient and any attempt to nurture it is good enough.

Reaching out for help

Anna's powerful story about the often unspoken experience of post-natal depression offers hope: there is light at the end of the tunnel. It is very common for mothers, like Anna, to struggle alone for a long time before seeking help. This is partly because they don't realise they need help, partly because they can be afraid to admit their feelings in case they are judged or, worse, have their baby taken from them. Seeking help and support is the most effective thing a mother can do.

Feeling alone and isolated is often as hard as any other aspect of PND. The old adage of 'a problem shared is a problem halved' is as applicable to PND as it is to any other area of life in which we may struggle. Your GP, or your public health nurse (PHN) may be the first person from whom to seek professional help. However, talking openly to your partner, parents or friends can make a difference.

Your GP may have different suggestions for treatment, including anti-depressants, which can be extremely useful. Counselling or therapy helps many mothers. There are lots of PND support groups in different areas of the country, and meeting other mothers who feel like you do can be really encouraging. If nothing else, it breaks the cycle of isolation and helps you to realise that the experience of depression is normal for others too.

Practical things you can do to reduce PND

Even if you don't seek professional help there are lots of things you can do to reduce the stress of parenting, and getting enough rest, especially in the early weeks and months, is vital. If all else fails, you can try the following:

* Agree with your partner that you have nights on and nights off to get up for your baby.
* If you are at home, try to take a nap whenever your baby sleeps. Never mind any chores; they can be left to your partner or will be easier when you've had some rest.
* Get regular fresh air and exercise; they help to build energy and make it easier to sleep when you have the chance.
* Ask friends and family to babysit regularly during the day

to allow you a few minutes, even an hour or two, to look after yourself (with a nap, a walk, or just a quiet cup of coffee).

✸ If someone offers help, always say yes.

Reducing exhaustion plays a significant role in helping the fog of PND to lift. It also helps to talk to other people about how you feel – at mother and baby groups, perhaps, in online discussion forums or with good friends and close relatives.

Don't forget to talk to your partner. If you feel able to confide in others, try to include your husband or partner in this. They may feel as bewildered as you do about being a parent, but may also be concerned about and confused by your mood, behaviour and attitude. They may feel helpless to intervene if you are withdrawn and uncommunicative; you may get more and better support if you share your experiences with them.

It may be tempting to compare yourself with other parents of small babies. However, we usually compare ourselves negatively and that doesn't help. The most common questions well-meaning people ask include: 'Does he sleep well for you?' or 'Is she a good baby?' How do you answer them? Babies are neither good nor bad; they are just babies, trying to communicate with us to have their needs met.

I came to resent that kind of question as it always made me feel I was being compared negatively to other parents, especially since our three babies had wonderfully chaotic and unsettled sleep patterns. I always felt an implied judgement in questions about sleep and believed I must be doing something wrong.

In my career subsequently I have come across such a huge variation in baby temperaments, sleep and crying patterns that I have realised there is no answer to such questions, or any need for one. Nonetheless, they always spark anxiety that we are not as successful in our parenting as others must be. They are best ignored when, in becoming a parent, your system has just withstood a tremendous shock.

PND can lift as long as we recognise it and try to do something about it. Reaching out and describing how you feel to someone you trust is the most important first step. Although PND might be a significant disruption to early family life, it will not prevent your family thriving as long as your baby's basic needs are met.

Understanding babies' crying

Babies' cries are the most heartbreaking, distressing, at times terrifying and often frustrating sounds to hear: Nature's warning system that a dependent infant needs attention. Whether it is about hunger, tiredness, discomfort from wee or poo, from being too hot or too cold or simply because they haven't been held for a while, your baby is trying to tell you something with their cry.

The question of 'spoiling'

Nature has created human babies to be helpless and entirely dependent on their parents. They can't do anything for themselves. Evolution requires families to nurture and protect their offspring. It makes best sense to me, therefore, for us to be responsive towards our babies. Responsiveness promotes secure attachment, which we know is a solid building block for thriving children.

Plenty of unsolicited advice may be offered by family and friends about whether to keep picking up your baby or not. But what does your gut tell you to do? Sometimes we worry that if we're too responsive we might 'spoil' our children. I'm sure we've all met children who appeared spoiled and overly entitled. These children have been appeased, and given in to, for many years. They have grown up believing that their demands, not only for what they need but also for what they want, will be met.

But infants don't cry for some wilful, unnecessary demand to be satisfied. They are not plotting and planning how to take advantage of their parents. If we employ kindness as a core value, then actually there is no dilemma: responding to your crying baby is simply the kindest thing to do. Moreover, it can be emotionally distressing for you and your baby to let him or her cry for extended periods.

Why babies cry

In babies, crying can serve several useful functions.

❋ It is a way to call for help when a baby is hungry, tired or uncomfortable.

❋ It helps to shut out other sounds or sights that may be over-stimulating, shocking or frightening.

❋ It helps to release tension, allowing a baby to reach a more settled state and sleep.

A case in point ...

John and Paula had an eighteen-week-old baby, Michael, when they contacted me for advice. They described how he had been in and out of hospital since birth; he had been admitted most recently at ten weeks old when he was taken critically ill. According to Paula, he was quite well again but had become used to either herself or John sitting by his cot day and night, a lot of the time holding his hand, and being there to comfort him constantly when doctors were putting in lines, etc.

The result of all this attention was that he still needed constant company and entertaining. When he couldn't see his mother or father he became anxious: his legs and arms started to flap and his breathing got much faster. Eventually he began crying. Given how sick he had been, Paula and John hated to see him cry and naturally assumed there was something seriously wrong with him. At the same time they were terrified that by attending to him every time he cried, they would spoil him.

Having listened to how worried they continued to be about his health, I reassured them that responding to him was the kindest and most natural thing they could do. Irrespective of his health, his cries carried meaning and the most important meaning was 'I need something'. Even if that need was company and comfort, it was worth responding so that their son could be secure in knowing that his parents were available to him.

As we spoke, John described another worry that their son wouldn't learn to entertain himself because he was so dependent on him and Paula. He was afraid that their baby would not become independent. Although in some ways his fears made sense, I reminded the couple that their baby was only four and a half months old and that independence of any description was a long way off.

It was interesting to hear John and Paula talking about their baby because the love and commitment they felt for him shone in every comment. They clearly loved him to bits. Despite that, they spoke about letting him cry it out so that he would learn to cope without them, because they felt they should be doing so. They sounded guilty, as if, by warmly responding to their baby, they were somehow treating him badly and destroying him for life. When I probed this conflict between what they instinctively felt they wanted to do (be responsive) and what they felt they should do (let him tough it out a bit), I started to hear the voice of John's mother.

John described his own upbringing in a family of five boys and one girl as a solid, no-nonsense experience. His mother and father were pragmatic people who just got on with things. They were warm but unfussy people, who rarely dwelled on their own or their children's emotional lives. As an example, he told me of an incident that had taken place when he was six and distraught at the loss of his favourite action figure, which he couldn't find. He went to his mother in floods of tears and was met with the simple statement that there were lots of other toys in the house to play with and that he was probably crying because he was hungry. He should come and have a bowl of soup. Now, twenty-five years later, she often commented on how lifting Michael so much would spoil him. 'There's no reason to go to him now; he's just winding you around his little finger. You've only just fed him so you need to leave him off now.'

Naturally, John believed his mum, who had raised six children, but felt the tug against some inner part of him that wanted to soothe his child. Interestingly, John's mother was not an unkind woman. When he had lost his action figure, his mother had responded in a way that was both nurturing and pragmatic (his upset may well have been exacerbated by hunger). I observed to John that her recent interventions seemed still to have his own best interests at heart, perhaps more than Michael's. She just wanted him not to be manipulated by his son. She didn't intend to be unkind to Michael; she just wanted John to have what she believed would be an easier time down the line.

Because Michael was so young, though, I felt his parents were not spoiling him by attending to him. I thought they were doing a good job, and that sticking by their instinct to be with him, to be gentle and responsive towards him, was good. Certainly there would come a time to set some limits and teach Michael that not everything would be done according to his demands, but not yet. For now, a kind, warm, responsive approach was what he needed.

The different meanings of a baby's cry

In the early weeks of family life none of us has a clue what needs an infant is expressing. It takes time for us to learn the differing tones they use. Their only way of expressing a need is to cry so we try to translate their cry and respond to our best guess as to what they need. For example, a hungry cry is usually short and low-pitched; it rises and falls. An angry cry tends to be more turbulent. A cry of pain or distress generally comes on suddenly and loudly, with a long, high-pitched shriek, followed by a pause, then a flat wail. The 'leave-me-alone' cry is usually similar to the hunger cry. It won't take long before you have a pretty good idea of what your baby's trying to tell you.

It's useful to remember that, in the early months, all of your baby's crying is healthy in that it serves a purpose for him or her. Sometimes different types of cry overlap. For example, newborns generally wake up hungry and crying for food. If you're not quick to respond, the hunger cry may give way to a wail of rage. You'll hear the difference. As your baby matures, her cries will become stronger, louder and more insistent. They'll also begin to vary more, as if to convey different needs.

Babies do cry to get noticed, which is no bad thing. Giving attention to small babies by responding to their cries for help will reduce the amount that they cry.

Responding to crying

Meeting the needs of our children is a fundamental part of parenting and central to a thriving family. It is a shame if adults don't meet those needs for comfort, security or reassurance because they're afraid of spoiling their infant. If you feel that your response to your baby or child is unkind, the chances are that a kinder response will be better emotionally for him or her – and for you.

As I explained to John and Paula when they came to talk to me, babies do learn to entertain themselves and can be separate from their parents, but usually for very brief periods before they return to the wonderfully powerful emotional and physical connection they have with us. At an early stage in babies' development, their contentment comes from their relationship with us so we need to invest heavily in responding to them when they need us.

It is important that we are not dissuaded from the belief that their crying is genuine. Sometimes we can feel we're being manipulated because this is what we're told. We need to understand that our babies lack the sophistication to manipulate us. They are simply doing what comes naturally.

Some ways to soothe crying babies

❃ Rocking them in your arms, on a rocking chair or in a crib

❃ Burping them in case they have trapped wind

❃ Talking gently and confidently to them (the tone of your voice is more important than what you say!)

❃ Singing lullabies or rhythmic, gentle tunes

❃ Gently massaging or stroking their tummy, head or back

❃ Wrapping them in a blanket to re-create the feeling of snugness from the womb

❃ Walking with them in your arms, a pram or baby sling

❃ Playing soft music (particularly music that you may have played during your pregnancy)

❃ Placing them close to the rhythmic sounds of a washing-machine (be wary of the spin cycle starting!) or a dishwasher

❃ Driving with them in the car when they are safely in their car seat

❃ Warm baths help some babies but not all.

Staying calm

The calmer we can remain when the baby is crying, the more successful we're likely to be at soothing them. Babies are very sensitive to tension and will often respond to it by crying. Listening to them can be agonising, though, and sometimes we need a break in order to be able to cope. No parent is ever able to console their baby all the time. Sometimes it helps to pass him or her to someone else for some relief and also because a new face and a different approach may help a baby to settle.

It can feel, at times, as if our babies are trying to get at us. It's important that we don't take their crying personally. They don't cry because they don't like us or because we're bad parents. Newborns can cry, for no apparent reason, for up to four hours a day. This is part of their adjustment to being in the world. Our own anger or impatience may build if we feel we're failing to settle them but it may help to remember that sometimes, no matter what we do, they may continue to cry. As long as we do our best to continue to respond we're doing enough.

Sensitively weaning a baby

When our babies are born we make a decision about whether to breast- or bottle-feed them. Whichever method we settle on, there will come a point when our baby needs to learn about other foods, tastes and textures. We call the process by which we slowly introduce new foods 'weaning'.

We may think that weaning is a short-term event, that we simply start giving new foods to our babies and that they quickly transfer from milk to solids. In fact, weaning is a long, slow process of letting a baby gently and consistently experience new foods in gradually increasing amounts.

Milk remains a crucial source of nutrition and comfort (because of the warm, close and nurturing associations a baby has with being fed milk). We need to resist the temptation to rush our baby through weaning; too much pressure to eat solid food may put him or her off it.

At the outset of weaning, babies' digestive systems are preparing to deal with more than milk so they can only cope with a very tiny amount of solid food. In many ways we can best think of their 'food' intake (separate from their milk intake) as being about exploring taste rather than nutrition.

Babies gain the bulk of their nutrition from milk. Milk has a much greater calorific content than an equivalent volume of puréed vegetables. A baby's stomach is the size of their closed fist; if they fill up with baby rice or puréed carrot, they won't take in all the calories they need for the growth and development they are engaged in. It may be up to eight months before a baby has a greater reliance on solid food than milk.

A case in point ...

Bridget contacted me about weaning sixteen-week-old Colm onto solids. He was a desperately hungry baby, she said, and his sleeping was terrible. She thought if she could get him onto solids he might settle better with a full tummy at night. By the time she met me it hadn't worked out that way. He was still waking and crying at night and he didn't seem to be as hungry for solid food as Bridget had expected. He hardly took any of the baby rice he was offered and turned his head away after the slightest taste. I remember Bridget saying to me, 'I feel desperate to get him to eat for me.'

As soon as I heard those words I was alerted to the likely source of the problem. Bridget was taking all the responsibility for Colm's eating, much as she had done when he was entirely dependent on milk. She wanted Colm to eat so that she could reduce her anxiety about his apparent hunger and the possibility that he was not getting enough food. She wanted him to eat so that he might feel full and satisfied enough to sleep through the night.

Bridget was missing the key point: weaning Colm onto solid food was a process of increasing his responsibility for what and how much he ate. Colm was giving her very clear messages that he was full enough by turning his head away and refusing the baby rice she offered. Understandably, Bridget probably assumed that he couldn't instinctively know how much food he needed and that his refusal was some kind of resistance to, or rejection of, her and her desire for him to eat.

The concept of Colm taking increasing responsibility for his solid-food intake formed the core of the work we did. Bridget and I discussed her own experiences of food. Unsurprisingly, she had grown up in a family that discouraged wasting food. She had been told to eat everything she was given because it was a sin to waste it, never mind the mantra about 'all the starving babies in Africa who don't have half of what you get'. Bridget had grown up eating out of a sense of duty. Leaving food was unconscionable for her. She detested waste. This dynamic, mixed with her fear about her son potentially starving to death if she didn't get enough food into him, led her to become very stressed about his apparently slow uptake of solid foods.

I insisted that Bridget be guided by his responses to the foods she offered him. If he turned his head away or spat out food, it meant that he'd had enough. It was really important that she didn't try to override this by forcing him to eat. All of the tricks and games we play with children at mealtimes, making 'aeroplanes' of spoons landing on the 'runway' of their mouths, are an attempt to cajole or persuade them to override the signals they are getting from their bodies. As I warned Bridget, this could lead Colm to a lifetime of misreading the physiological signals.

The main lesson that Bridget took away, she told me later, was that Colm was eating because he needed the food and that it was okay for him to determine how much he ate at any sitting. Essentially, she had realised he could become responsible for deciding what he ate. She had seen weaning him onto solids as a tool to fill and settle him at night. She hadn't appreciated that weaning is about allowing children to become more responsible.

This revolutionised her approach to Colm's mealtimes. She became more patient with him and recognised that sometimes he would be hungry for solids and at others he might not and that either was okay. She stopped stressing about the volume of solids he consumed and allowed him more control over holding his spoon or food and attempting to feed himself (a messy procedure that left most of the food on the high chair and the floor!). She told me, laughing, at our three-month review that his sleeping was still a disaster but she cared less about it now because they enjoyed their mealtimes so much more.

> ## Cajoling children into eating can create resistance
>
> Pleading with, cajoling and forcing children to eat what they don't want can produce such stress in them that it can be counterproductive. Rather than learning to eat a balanced diet, they build up resistance to certain foods and mealtimes because they associate them with so much stress.

Introducing solids

Ideally, we want our children to experience food as nurturing. Given how important it is to our health, it is also a cornerstone to thriving in its most physical sense. The relationship that children have with food is influenced and guided from the first attempts we make to wean them. Giving them responsibility for what they eat is one of the great gifts we can bestow on them.

A healthy attitude to food will protect them from over- and under-eating. More importantly, though, responsibility for what they eat is part of the overall sense of responsibility that children need to acquire. Eating is a behaviour and, like all other behaviours, we will be accountable for it in adulthood. Ideally we will send our children the right message from the start.

A baby has an instinctive desire to eat. Their only difficulty is that in infancy they can't go and get food for themselves. They have to hope that the right kind of food is presented to them. At this stage, they can't be fully responsible for what they eat. We must be responsible for ensuring they strike the right balance between milk and solid food. We must also ensure that children get what they need in a timely fashion.

If we cling to the control of food, though, and try to insist they eat a particular amount or type of food, we will quickly overwhelm any natural choices a baby might make about whatever we have offered. If this is a child's experience of weaning, they may never learn to make food choices (other than, perhaps, refusing to eat what they're presented with!). We want our children to thrive, and ensuring that they eat well is part of that. A responsive approach to weaning that allows babies to decide how much or little they eat sets the tone for a thriving attitude to food.

Sleep and getting enough of it

Sleeping is a huge issue for families, and parents get very stressed, and utterly exhausted, if their babies and children have consistently disrupted sleep. It is hard not to be short-tempered and resentful if we're disturbed at night. If wakefulness occurs regularly, parents will inevitably become exhausted and grumpy, which may have an impact on all other areas of family life.

A common sleeping myth

The myth that it is normal for infants to sleep through the night circulates regularly, adding to parental stress. New families can feel under major pressure to have their baby in some fabulous night-time routine that involves twelve hours of uninterrupted sleep. In my experience, it is rarely that simple. In my practice I have heard of every combination of how much and where babies and children sleep. Certainly for infants, it is more normal to wake periodically through the night, since at the very least they need to feed.

The need for comfort and security

Even in adulthood we can find ourselves lying awake for ages, unable to fall sleep. Sometimes worries keep us awake, with thoughts and feelings tumbling around and our brains refusing to switch off. The shape or firmness of a strange mattress, a too-hot or too-cool room, may mean we find it hard to get comfy. Children and babies are no different.

When we were small our mothers and/or fathers probably tried to create the most comfortable environment for us to sleep in. That may have meant they stayed with us while we drifted off (to give us that sense of security). Maybe we shared a room with a sibling (or two or three). Maybe our parents left a light on, or the door open, and checked us often to make sure we were okay.

At some point, though, we learned to soothe ourselves to sleep. We no longer relied on our parents to help us feel secure and comfortable, having developed those resources within ourselves. This is a phase that every child must go through. As a parent we can decide to wean children gently off the need for our support (my preferred approach) or opt for a 'cold turkey' approach: then parents leave their child to cry themselves to sleep.

Typical sleep habits of babies

Small babies need to sleep for between twelve and fifteen hours in a 24-hour period; when they are between six and twelve weeks old, most of them will have slotted into a clear day/night rhythm and take the majority of their sleep at night. In an ideal world, therefore, a baby will sleep for ten to twelve hours through the night, with the remainder taken in a couple of naps during the day. But the world is rarely ideal!

Babies have a sleep cycle that moves from drifting off to sleep, then falling into a deep sleep and back to rapid eye movement sleep (REM sleep). The cycle can take anything between twenty and about forty minutes. When babies and children wake up, it is usually during an REM period because that is when our brains are back to being active, even though we remain asleep. We think that dreaming occurs in the REM period of each cycle. In an eleven-hour night, most babies will go through between fifteen and twenty such cycles. Some babies will wake up every time they hit an REM period.

Helping children to soothe themselves to sleep

We need to be able to sleep and we need to teach our children to soothe themselves to sleep. There are two key elements in this: helping them to fall asleep on their own, then getting them to soothe themselves back to sleep rather than calling for help.

My preferred approach, without damaging trust or emotionally traumatising a baby, is to wean him or her slowly and gently off their reliance on us to soothe them. In this way they learn that we're available to help them regulate their anxieties or give comfort, but that they don't necessarily need us to provide that. Rather, they find the resources to meet those needs for themselves. Crucially, however, they know that we are reliably on hand if they do need us.

Stages of gently teaching children to settle themselves

1. Developing a consistent bedtime routine

Typically, newborn babies often fall asleep in our arms while they're being fed. Equally, if they're being rocked or cuddled they may drift off. It comes as a big shock to them when they wake in a cot or a crib with no warm adult. No wonder they scream! When children fall asleep in the same location as they wake up, they are not so surprised and do not find the transition from wakefulness to sleep to wakefulness so upsetting.

It helps if a baby gets used to a consistent sleep environment; he or she can begin to develop a sense of comfort and security from being put down, falling asleep and waking in a way that is familiar, understood and predictable. They come to make comforting associations with the colours, sounds and textures of their room and cot.

A full bedtime routine often includes a last feed taken downstairs, a good burp, a bath, a fresh nappy, a Babygro, and being laid in his or her cot. Then we might read a story, sing a lullaby, say prayers and place a reassuring hand on their tummy.

2. Shifting any association between feeding and sleeping

Shifting an association that a baby has developed between feeding and falling asleep is an important first step in teaching him or her to settle themselves at night. As long as babies are fed to get them to sleep at the start of the night, they will maintain an association between feeding and falling asleep to the extent that they will expect a feed whenever they wake. However, given how much physical comfort most babies receive from feeding, we invariably find that we still have to be physically present with our baby at this stage to substitute for feeding.

So, when you're ready to make this change, you'll give your baby their last evening feed before starting the bedtime routine. If they seem to be dozing, or are about to fall asleep, interrupt the feed to ensure that they don't drop off too soon. When the feed is finished, you can wind them, and continue to prepare them for bed.

As with any transition, it takes time for babies to become accustomed to the change. It may take up to a month for your baby to settle without a feed at bedtime. It can really help to stay close to your baby, keeping a hand on her, for physical reassurance, while she gets used to sleeping without feeding. In the early stages of weaning a baby off milk at night, they require a heavy investment of our time and presence to soothe them.

3. Reducing your physical contact while they fall asleep

Assuming you have physically comforted your baby while they fall asleep, the next step is to begin to withdraw your physical touch as they drop off. Your baby will probably still get upset without being held, so for a number of nights we may need to remain very close and perhaps continue to stroke their tummy occasionally, hum or talk warmly to them until they settle or fall asleep. Even if your baby is crying, the key is to stay close by and do your best to comfort them, but relying on less physical contact to do so.

If your baby gets really distressed, consistently, then he or she may be telling you that they are not ready for this stage and you may choose to return to the previous stage of holding or rocking them to sleep for a week or so before trying again.

Within a short period of time, though, most babies realise that we are still nearby and still willing to soothe them with a quick tummy rub; they stop protesting and get used to falling asleep. We need to give them at least a week to get established in this new routine of being in their cot with little or no touching before we move to the next step.

4. Withdrawing your physical touch entirely

The next step is to stop touching your baby at all as he or she lies in the cot. You can continue to stay very near and to make occasional comforting sounds. Most babies, by this stage, will be satisfied by your presence alone and settle quickly into this new habit. Again, give your baby at least a week to get used to you being present but not touching them before taking the final step.

5. Slowly withdrawing from the room while your baby falls asleep

The last step is to begin to withdraw altogether. We start by staying in the room all the time, but at a distance from the cot. Over time, we move just outside the door, but checking in on the baby regularly.

Finally, once we're outside the room we need to keep returning regularly to check on the baby so that he or she can be reassured that we're still in the building! Over time we can increase the period between checking visits until we reach the point when we can give our baby a last kiss goodnight and leave them to fall asleep entirely unaided.

At each of these stages we allow our babies to settle into the new rhythm before moving to the next stage. Unremarkably, when they learn to fall asleep alone, at the start of the night, we find that they can fall back to sleep alone if they wake during the night. So, over a period of a couple of months or so, we can move from feeding a baby to sleep, and having to get up to them several times in the night, to having uninterrupted sleep ourselves and a contented sleeping baby.

The question of allowing babies to cry themselves to sleep

Crying it out can be very distressing for babies and parents. Emotionally, a child who falls asleep alone and distraught will feel that nobody cared about him or her because nobody responded. I think this is traumatising for a small child or an infant. Some schools of thought may suggest that babies need to learn to cry and then to cope on their own, but if you stick with what we know about babies expressing their needs by crying, then night crying needs a response. If we try to toughen a child up by letting him or her cry, I believe it may damage their core ability to trust adults. It's well worthwhile taking the time to teach our babies how to settle themselves, as described above.

A case in point ...

George and Amanda were first-time parents who came to see me about their eight-month-old daughter, Julie, and her sleeping (or lack of it). They said she had great difficulty getting to sleep in the first place and couldn't stay asleep or resettle herself if she woke (sometimes up to eight times a night).

Amanda breastfed Julie, and always to get her to sleep. When Julie woke, she wouldn't be soothed by George and only settled with Amanda if she fed her again. George and Amanda described themselves as 'walking zombies' through the days, such was their exhaustion. They were constantly rowing and were at loggerheads over how to deal with Julie's sleep.

I empathised with their plight. Indeed, as a parent of three breastfed children I could also sympathise with the terrible tiredness and the grumpy, short-tempered sniping between husband and wife. We all want children to sleep better but first we have to understand why they wake and how we can coax them back to sleep. It seemed to help George and Amanda to understand that waking regularly is not uncommon with babies and children, especially breastfed babies. Lots of babies rely on the comfort and security of sucking a breast to help them fall asleep.

It was only natural, therefore, that when their daughter wanted comfort to drift off to sleep she looked to feed for emotional and physical wellbeing. From her point of view, as long as she was feeding, all was well in her world. This reassured both parents as it normalised their family experience and helped them understand that there was nothing wrong with Julie or them.

The solution for George and Amanda, I felt, was either to continue to provide the comfort and security that breastfeeding offered at night or gently wean Julie from night feeding while also weaning her from reliance on her parents to soothe her to sleep. Determined to reclaim their sleep, George and Amanda opted to wean Julie according to my guidelines. Over the next couple of months I supported them as they worked through the process.

Of course there were blips along the way. Julie took her time in accepting that she wasn't going to be fed to sleep, so it took a few weeks of one or other parent being near her cot whenever she woke. Interestingly, George became as successful as Amanda at settling Julie once the demand for and expectation of breast milk was reduced.

Once she had learned to fall asleep alone at the start of the night she was also able to settle back to sleep, if she woke in the middle of the night, without calling to her parents. Although the whole process took about four months, the family reached a peaceful bedtime and enjoyed nights with no distress, or damaged trust, for anyone.

Getting older children to sleep in their own bed

The staged weaning process is exactly the same approach that I take to moving children into their own bed if they have been previously bed-sharing or co-sleeping with us. Co-sleeping (having children in the same room as their parents) is another powerful way to give children a strong certainty that their needs will be reliably met, at night, by their parents. It aids the establishment of trust between us and our children, but eventually we want our space back!

It would be a shame to shift a child suddenly into their own room without support. That kind of change could be destabilising and distressing. Making it a gentle, gradual process will show us to be reliable and won't affect the trust that has built up between us and our child. We can use our presence while they fall asleep as a bridge for them in the transition to their own bed. Then over time we can slowly withdraw as they learn confidently to settle alone.

Helping parents and babies to cope with separation anxiety

The most significant separation that many mothers and babies face is the return to work after maternity leave. For fathers it may have occurred sooner. However, there are many other smaller separations, such as when we leave our babies with their granny, a friend, even our partner, and they have to cope without us. If, and when, babies fret at a parent's absence we call it separation anxiety.

Understanding why babies protest at our absence

Separation anxiety is natural and to be expected. Children protest at the initial separation because they are upset by the 'loss' of their parent and worry instinctively about how they will cope without them. Babies miss us and may 'panic' at not having the usual reassurance and comfort from us. They get upset on the parent's return perhaps as a way of saying, 'I'm cross with you for leaving me,' and also, perhaps, because they feel relief at our return and, unconsciously, no longer feel the need to cope without us.

It makes sense, too, that your baby will have become reliant on you to meet their emotional needs. This is the very dynamic that we have tried to build by being so responsive to them. If you have had four, six, eight months or more with your baby, you have probably built a wonderfully secure attachment and have allowed your baby to be appropriately reliant on you. You have shown yourself to be trustworthy.

It is undeniably a wrench for you and your baby if you can no longer provide that continuity. It is also a fact of life for many families. How we manage the separation, supporting our babies in getting used to the new arrangements, says a lot about our core understanding of babies' needs and what we believe to be important about family relationships.

The clingy baby

Clinginess is not necessarily a sign of insecure attachment. It indicates that a child may feel unsure of their surroundings and wants their parent to help them regulate their emotions. Most securely attached infants and toddlers will cling to their parent at times of stress or threat. An insecurely attached child may also be clingy but they are less likely to allow themselves to be settled or calmed by their parent. They may remain fussy and whingey and may not let go of us, even though they don't settle well with us. Securely attached children trust us to keep them safe! Once the threat passes or they become used to a situation, they usually feel confident to explore further from their parent, with the occasional return to closeness, just for reassurance.

How trust is transferred in babies

When we have invested in creating a trusting relationship with our child, we can assume that he or she is going about their day feeling very content and knowing they can rely on us. It also means that they will look at most adults and assume they will provide the equivalent care too. If they trust us, they have probably no reason, yet, not to trust others. Once children have experienced at least one secure attachment to a parent (or both) it frees them to develop further secure and confident relationships.

If we have been at home with an infant for many months, we may worry that the strength of their connection to us means they will feel the effect of a separation more (and they might), but it also means that they will have the resilience and capacity to form secure and trusting relationships with others (especially their new childminder).

How babies' anxieties are linked to our own

Babies usually take their cues on how to behave, and even how to feel, from others around them. We can see this when they bump their heads and, rather than crying instantly, look around to gauge the reaction of their parents. If they see us smiling and saying cheerfully, 'Bumps-a-daisy, all fall down,' or something like that, they may smile in response rather than focusing on the hurt.

Equally, if we seem distressed or worried in a given situation our baby will tune in to our anxiety. Many parents get very worried at the prospect of leaving their baby; if we seem worried our baby will assume there is something to be worried about and show signs of distress. Unfortunately this can become circular: the more distressed the baby becomes, the more distressed we become . . .

For much the same reason, though, a baby is likely to take his or her emotional lead from whichever adult is caring for them when we aren't there. As long as their childminder is stable, confident, warm and caring, a baby will feel supported and, even if they're upset at our absence, will allow themselves to be comforted by their new carer. All of our investment in building trust through security of attachment means that our babies can trust their childminder to take care of them too.

A case in point ...

June was a full-time mother to sixteen-month-old Rory. He had suffered badly with infant reflux until just before she came to meet me. June had breastfed him until he was a little over a year old and told me that he had never left her side, day or night, through his first year. She had never left him with grandparents or family because he couldn't be settled. She wondered if he was now so incredibly dependent on her for security that it would cause him great emotional trauma and anxiety if she left him.

She said he was desperately clingy and got very upset any time she tried to leave him with his granny, to the point that she always changed her plans and stayed with him or took him with her.

I was intrigued by June's comment that nobody else could settle Rory during his first year. She didn't even feel that his dad could calm him. When we talked more about this, it turned out that she had never really trusted anyone else to calm him so had never given anyone an opportunity to try. Indeed, even now when she was due to leave him with her mother, she became very anxious. It was June's own fears of letting Rory go that we ended up focusing on.

Together we traced back June's childhood experiences of trust. As I had expected, she had always felt insecure. Her insecurity had grown from the particularly high expectations that her parents had had of her when she was growing up. June had always thought she failed to meet the standard set by her parents and had never felt she was good enough. An underlying anxiety about not meeting expectations, not doing well enough, not being perfect is often expressed in parenting by over-protectiveness. Never mind our children clinging to us, we cling to them because, at heart, we worry about how they will survive in the world. Our fears at letting them go may sometimes be a significant block.

As a consequence, the letting-go process for June was daunting and she dreaded it. The process of adjustment, or accommodation, to this change in her relationship with Rory (she would no longer be his only carer) was a huge deal for her. As with many other parents, the first step in dealing with the separation was for her to try to understand and regulate her feelings about letting go.

I encouraged her to express her worries about missing him and about whether he would cope with her mother and her husband. That way, she was less likely to transfer her worries to Rory – a crucial step. I expected June to get feedback from her mum and husband about whether her anxieties seemed normal, or whether they veered into irrational and overprotective, which might hamper Rory's confidence to be in the world.

Once June understood her emotional world better, she was able to move to the practical preparations for letting Rory go. First, she arranged visits to her mum, with Rory, while she remained present, and saw how warmly and lovingly her mum interacted with him. Reassured, she then used the visits as an opportunity to go out for short periods, giving her baby practice at being without her and also letting him learn that after a time she always returned. This took a while but allowed June and Rory both to establish trust in the world as a safe enough place, to understand that they could survive without each other and look forward to the reunion.

Familiarity with a new situation reduces anxiety

Taking a staged approach to leaving your baby with a new minder or crèche is common sense. The more babies and children know about what to expect, the more predictable their world becomes. When things are predictable for children, they are less anxious. So, spending an hour in the crèche, with you, allows them to feel safe in the new place, supported by you. Next time you can chance leaving them for an hour without you. Returning to collect them, dependably and consistently, also helps them to predict the experience of being with another carer.

When babies and children can see that we interact warmly and confidently with a new person, they understand that they, too, can be confident in the new person. So, for example, when I meet new clients I always spend time talking with their parents so that the child can see that their parent feels safe and secure in my company. This helps the child with their early decisions about whether they will be safe and secure with me.

Sometimes it may also help a child to keep with them some comfort item from home, like a stuffed toy or a blankie, as it provides some continuity and comfort in the absence of their parent.

Coping with tears at separation time

Children crying at a separation can rock our faith in their ability to be okay, and our own ability to cope, when we're parted from each other. Challenging as it can be, we need to try not to seem bothered if our baby cries as we leave them. It's simply their survival instinct kicking in: 'Don't leave me! I rely on you for everything – how am I going to cope without you?' It's designed, very determinedly, to keep us present by making us feel guilty and torn about going.

The reality, of course, is that within a very short space of time, usually a few minutes, the same instinct reminds him or her to make the best of the situation as it is so they just get on with the new arrangements. If they can thrive at home with us, they will thrive in most circumstances where they are treated kindly and responsibly.

Once they have had time to adjust and gain confidence and trust in whoever is minding them, they stop fussing so much when we go: leaving us and going to the childminder (or the crèche) becomes a transition from one secure base to another.

Thriving from the start of family life

So many of the issues that we face in the early days, weeks and months of our parenting careers are entirely new and we have no script, or previous experience, to draw on. As a consequence we rely on our intuition, what feels right or best to do. Often this fits with what our baby needs. We also draw on advice from extended family, friends and books like this one. Often the advice we receive from different sources can conflict with our own beliefs, and our advisers' suggestions may be in conflict with each other. We then have to decide on what approach or response seems most closely to match the values we hold true.

Ultimately we are only ever trying to do the best we can. There is no perfect way to respond to our babies. As long as our core sense is to be responsive and warm, we are likely to offer them good enough care to feel secure and nurtured. If we hold them close when they are babies, there will be plenty of time to let them go a little, towards their ultimate independence, when they are older.

03
THRIVING THROUGH THE TODDLER AND PRESCHOOL YEARS

Active engagement: the true mark of the toddler

In the toddler and pre-school years, adult reliability remains crucial, but this is when children first establish their separateness. Toddlers, who are testing the boundaries of their expanding world, will present new challenges to parents, and the dynamic of family life can be significantly altered. Instead of being comparatively passive recipients, as infants are, of parental care and attention, toddlers become very active participants in, and explorers of, their environment.

Exploration through trial and error

Small children explore their world in a very physical way. Everything is tried and tested. Trial and error is the somewhat clumsy but only approach open to small children. In theory, the consequences of their actions are important since this is how they learn. If, for example, they pull a pot out of the cupboard and it slides out easily to become the perfect drum, they are likely to return to the cupboard every time they feel like banging the pot. If, however, in pulling the pot out they displace a larger pile of pots that crashes noisily to the floor and they get a fright, they might think twice about pulling out another pot, or even refuse to do so.

In their trials and tribulations, however, they are essentially self-centred and little concerned about the needs of others. A toddler will happily grab a piece of cake without considering whether anyone else might like it. If he or she sees a toy they want, they will take it, even if another child is playing with it. They may only stop to wonder if they are strong enough to wrest it from the other child.

Remaining calm and understanding in the aftermath of their experimentation requires, at times, unlimited patience and goodwill.

The challenge to authority

For families this can be the stage at which the first serious battles for power and control are fought. Toddlers and pre-schoolers just want their own way and parents often find themselves at odds as they try to manage their toddler's behaviour to keep them safe and to ensure that family life meets the needs of every member.

Toddlers love to say, 'No.' It can seem to many of us that this is the first and only word they use! We may feel affronted by their apparent opposition, no matter what we suggest or ask of them. However, saying 'No', or being oppositional, is a natural part of their developing separateness. In the toddler years children first begin the process of individuation, i.e. becoming individuals. In their infancy, babies consider themselves and their primary carer to be one being, indivisible. As they reach toddlerhood they realise they are separate beings and, almost to underline that separateness, try to show themselves to be different from their carers.

Individuation is an ongoing process throughout the rest of their childhood and adolescence. We usually feel it most strongly again in their teenage years as they fully separate and become independent of us. Adolescence is often the next biggest challenge to our authority.

Consequently, we need not panic at our toddler's seeming bolshie: this is part of their developmental work and is why this period is often referred to as the 'terrible twos'. How we respond to their tantrums, refusals and frustrations will often determine the tone of family life and set a pattern for our interaction with them for years to come. This is the time when we have to introduce firmness into our relationship with them. Crucially, though, we need to moderate it with lots of kindness.

Setting the tone with firm but kind discipline

The theme of discipline, and how to discipline, is often first expressed during this period in family life. As ever, we must have an eye to the past because the influences of our own parents and how they disciplined us will be beacons to our engagement with our children. We need to set limits and guide our toddlers' behaviour. We still have to determine and regulate most of what they do, showing backbone ourselves. Achieving this without becoming angry, or over-punitive, is a real challenge for parents who can feel pushed to the pin of their collar by these obstinate, wilful, belligerent, yet adorable forces of nature. Remembering that they are good children who occasionally do bold things may help us to remain kind and considerate towards them.

Learning to share

Negotiating with and adjusting to the rights and needs of others are tough jobs. Attending crèches and pre-schools involves children in learning to live among an arbitrary social group of their peers for several hours each day. The role of the family, to me, is as important as the work of the crèche leaders in determining how successful this will be for individual children. Teaching children to share is the start of teaching them that other children (and adults) have needs and feelings.

When they realise that someone else wants the same toy, or is upset if it is grabbed from them, it is a sign that they can see the world from someone else's perspective. This is really hard for small children to achieve and so, initially, we teach them to share by rote learning. We worry less that they understand why they must share and more that they actually do share. We, at times physically, guide and direct their behaviour to give a toy to another child or take their turn with it.

Sometimes consideration of others is first experienced within families as the adults and the child must find a means of accommodating themselves to a second and subsequent children. Making space, literally, for a new baby is a common enough experience for toddlers and most of them don't like it. While they may tolerate an immobile infant, a ten-month-old brother or sister who can crawl into the middle of their game and disrupt it is much less welcome. However, understanding the frustrations of jealous toddlers means we can be more patient in helping them to build tolerance and become inclusive.

The importance of learning patience

Our children's growth into toddlerhood, especially their increasing autonomy, means that we also have to shift our expectations of what we do as parents. The tasks of parenting in babyhood are very much about providing physical and emotional care. We don't have to instruct babies. All of our warm and considerate interactions with them will teach them about a range of things, like trust, reliability and language.

In the toddler years, we are more instructive, as well as simply being with our children. This is our first opportunity to teach them about our values and beliefs. As our children learn language we can interact with them in a whole new way. They understand our verbal instructions and can respond to give us more insight into their inner world of thoughts and feelings. Sometimes, though, we can be duped into thinking they are more advanced than they are and have unrealistically high expectations of them.

They may not fully understand all of a complex two- or three-part direction, for example. They may not be able to organise themselves to put on their own shoes. They may not remember to share, or that it isn't okay to bite in frustration. They may not have the patience to wait in the shop, or at the dinner table. So, while we want to show them the best way to interact successfully in the world, we need to remember that they are still very young and will make lots of mistakes. We often have to take a deep breath, grit our teeth, smile and have another go.

Thriving through the toddler years takes lots of time, energy and patience. But responding to a toddler's behaviour in a consistent, firm and understanding way will allow them to grow from a very solid base.

How play connects us with our children

Play is an essential and natural activity for children; it stimulates their brains. They explore and discover their world through play. They communicate feelings through play. They work through stressful situations and relieve tension when they play, and they also use it as an opportunity to spend time and develop connections with the people they care about.

Let's be honest, we love having other children round to play because it can be a great distraction for our own children. Once they have settled together, we can catch up on other things around the house while keeping an occasional eye on what they're up to. However, if we want to use play to connect with our children and build a thriving relationship with them, we have to be involved in it to a greater or lesser extent.

Free-play

Free-play is unstructured time for a child when they can choose the objects and situations they want to play with. When a child plays freely they are fully in charge of what they do. During free-play, a child decides how and what they want to play, according to their desires, imagination and ability. Many parents rely on their children taking lots of free-play time. Indeed, it can often suit us to have our children playing independently of us as it frees us to do other jobs. But we need to make sure we're letting them play freely for their benefit and not just for our own!

Involving ourselves in children's play

Dads, especially, have a habit of involving themselves in their children's play, then taking over. We love to dictate how toys should be played with or constructed. When you watch some dads playing with their children, you realise that the dads are playing and the children are spectating or have become distracted elsewhere. Ideally we would take this as an indication that we need to do things differently! Our children's voices and actions must be heard and recognised in their own play.

Sometimes, though, we have to provide support to them; they may be finding something hard to do or want our help or company. The kind of support that allows a child to play as they like, but with a bit of help to make it work, is called 'scaffolding'. Figuratively, we are providing the scaffold within which they construct the game or the play scenario. Sometimes we offer suggestions or guidance, sometimes physical help. Importantly, though, parents are not trying to take over or structure the play in a particular way. Rather, we are providing the help and encouragement that a child needs to pursue their own ideas or objectives.

Determining our children's play

At other times adults can structure the playtime. This means that the adult decides the types of games a child or children will play. Sometimes children find it easier to have a clear set of instructions about what to do and how to do it, particularly if they are unsure or anxious about what is expected of them. For example, a young child is going to a play-date with a friend. If the friend's house is unfamiliar, the visiting child may not be sure what to expect. A parent getting involved early in the children's play may ease the transition, allowing them to get used to the house and being with their friend, and have them playing co-operatively from the outset.

Games with rules are a very structured form of play, although small children may not always stick to the rules! Rules specify how a game should be played, to ensure fairness and to identify how games start, proceed and finish, including how somebody wins. When rules are applied (and enforced) in games, the play can become predictable. Children can learn to trust that they will be treated fairly and that it will be their skill at the game (with some luck usually) that will be the deciding factor in winning or losing.

This maintenance of their faith in 'fair play' is why children often become so focused on the application of rules. In contrast, their desire to win may lead them to become focused on adapting, changing or ignoring the rules to suit themselves. Small children find it really hard to lose, so only some of their games should be competitive. Any game that has winners and losers is competitive. Learning to cope with losing is a life lesson and can be good, but only if adults are there to help the child to understand and regulate their disappointment.

Learning about sharing and turn-taking

There is a real opportunity for parents to be instructive during playtime. When it comes to sharing and turn-taking, play is an ideal opportunity to teach children about considering the needs of others. Co-operative play is quite challenging for toddlers and pre-schoolers to achieve. When you look at small children playing in a group you will discover that, in the main, they are engaged in parallel play: they are playing alongside other children but separately from them. There is normally very little overlap between the activities of various children. Sharing and turn-taking are skills that are essential to co-operative play but most toddlers have not yet learned them.

Non-competitive play ideas

You will find lots more in an Internet search.

* Any kind of craft activity
* Water or sand
* Play with action figures, animals or dolls
* Doing puzzles
* Collecting leaves or bark rubbings
* Building forts indoors or outdoors.

Non-competitive game ideas

Again, search the Internet for more ideas.

* **Keep It Up** – work together to keep a balloon in the air.
* **Co-operative Musical Chairs** – the children have to help each other: they make space to squeeze onto chairs together or sit on each other's knees as successive chairs are removed at each round.
* **Mirror-mirror** – the children have to mimic the actions of the leader.
* **Simon Says** – the children have to follow the verbal instructions of a leader; it is played co-operatively when nobody is out if they make a mistake.
* **Chain Tag** – played with one person 'on'; as they tag other children, they join hands to make an increasingly long chain of 'on' children.

Toddlers don't choose to take turns with a ball. They will play with it until they are tired of it or distracted by some other toy that grabs their fancy. So, in the case of a play-date where two boys are together, an adult will have to step in to ensure that their child gives a turn with the ball to the other boy and that the other boy then returns the favour. This might mean sitting between them and suggesting, 'Now you roll the ball to Billy, and Billy, you roll the ball back to Johnny.' You may even have to prompt one or both boys physically to roll the ball to the other.

This activity gives each child the experience of letting the ball go and learning that it gets given back. Because the adult is structuring this and ensuring fairness in the sharing, each boy can learn to trust a little more in the concept of sharing. They learn essentially that 'what goes around, comes around': if you give to others, they give back to you.

How children create structured play with their peers

If you listen to older children creating imaginative play scenarios with their friends, you will hear them creating rules and structure for the game. A seven-year-old boy may say, 'We'll both be heroes and I'll have the sword of strength to give me my fighting power. You'll have the bow and arrow that never misses as your power. But you can't shoot if the enemies are too close so that'll be my job.' His fellow hero may add, 'Yeah, and my arrows can go through armour but your sword will only go through skin so in the battles you have to leave the armoured demons for me to kill.'

The rest of their imaginary battle will be played out according to their agreed rules about their powers and abilities, and the success of the game will depend on them sticking to the rules. Often we find that successful pairings on play-dates are those friends who can trust each other to stick to the agreed plan.

Somewhere along the way those children have learned important messages about trust, usually from adult intervention in their play.

They have learned to stick to their word and the rules so that the game is fair and enjoyable for all.

A case in point ...

Paul and his wife, Imelda, had one child, a boy named Jonathan, who was four. Jonathan was having a difficult time in pre-school and was regularly in trouble for being out of his seat, distracting other children, fighting in the playground, interrupting other children's games and generally making a nuisance of himself. As I explored these issues with Paul and Imelda, I discovered that Jonathan was also very testing at home. He regularly opposed any correction by his parents, but seemed particularly cross with Paul. He often said things to Paul like, 'You're not the boss of me,' and on a few occasions had even told Paul to 'Fuck off and leave me alone.'

Several things struck me about how out of control Jonathan's behaviour seemed to be. The most significant was how ill-disciplined he was. He accepted no structure or limits from his parents (or teacher) and chose to do exactly as he liked. Neither Paul nor Imelda seemed very able or willing to challenge this. The focus of my work became empowering the couple to take charge. Also, Paul and Imelda needed to prove themselves reliable and trustworthy so that Jonathan would know that if they said something they would follow through on it.

I decided to use play as the means to empower the family. I got each of the parents to play with Jonathan separately and together. I showed them what to do and encouraged them to invest a lot of time, positively, in being with Jonathan and structuring his play. I wanted them to provide some rules for the games and, most importantly, to enforce them. Their intention was not to be punitive if Jonathan broke the rules, but to praise him every time he followed them and enjoyed the game.

Jonathan took a bit of time to get into the habit of playing with his parents because they had never really spent time with him in that way before. However, after some initial resistance and disruption of the games, Jonathan began to respond to their relentlessly positive attitude towards the play and their praise and encouragement of him when he engaged in the games.

Within a few weeks a number of important things had shifted for the family. First, they had got to know each other better and their relationships with each other had improved because they were spending more time together. Second, Jonathan had begun to accept the notion of rules and learned that he could trust his parents to be fair in upholding them. He also learned that his parents were not afraid to say, 'No,' to him in the midst of play and that, actually, he could accept it and still enjoy himself. Without any of them noticing, the same dynamic began to emerge in daily life. Jonathan enjoyed his parents' company more and they found themselves being more assertive about what was okay and not okay in terms of his behaviour.

I had reckoned that Jonathan was particularly angry with Paul because he missed him; Paul kept very long hours at work. But because Paul and Imelda invested more time in play with Jonathan, Paul, especially, had become much more available to his son. Consequently, Jonathan no longer had to show his dad that he was cross with him for being away so much and his challenging behaviour diminished. By playing with their son, Paul and Imelda also showed him that they noticed him, cared about him and wanted to be with him, all of which added to Jonathan's growing trust in his parents and led to a huge reduction in his challenging behaviour at home and, in due course, at school too.

The extra benefits of having fun with your children

I'm always warmed when I think of this family because their story shows so clearly how investing time in playing with your child can dramatically improve your relationship with them. Of course it was important how they played with him, but it didn't really matter what they played. The key elements that built a positive relationship were:

* The games had rules.
* The rules were fairly applied.
* The family focused more on the fun and enjoyment of playing than the winning and losing.
* The parents were able empathetically to acknowledge their son's disappointment if he lost.
* The parents were firm but fair in keeping the structure of the game together.

The dynamic this created transformed the relationships between Jonathan and his parents. Where once there was conflict, distrust and disrespect, now they had started to thrive in an engaged, fun way.

The role of horseplay and wrestling in play

I especially love a game with my children that involves horseplay. I find it wonderfully instructive, and it allows us all to let off excess energy. I call it 'tumble-time' or sometimes the 'rolly-tumbly-monster game'. It's a variation on wrestling! I use it with my children for fun but also when there's frustration in the air. I find that play-wrestling helps to vent some of my children's troublesome feelings and allows me to re-establish myself as a dad who is in charge both practically and emotionally.

I set up the game with two rules. First, no hurting is allowed. Second, if anyone says stop, we stop immediately. After that, no holds are barred. When we play, which we do on my bed, I still feel I'm in charge because I'm the adult determining whether my child is 'winning' by overcoming me or whether I'm 'winning' by overcoming them. Depending on the situation, I can let both or either scenario develop.

If you allow a child to appear more powerful than you for a short while, they may gain a sense of satisfaction, which helps to build their confidence. In a tough, long-drawn-out tussle, a child can work off energy that might otherwise be directed harmfully at a sibling! Also, while they're in mid-exertion, I can name some of their frustrations, which often leads to a renewed physical struggle that helps to resolve the problem. For example, I may say, 'I think you hate it when I tell you what to do. You'd love to be let do whatever you want.' This kind of statement is often met with a shout of rage and a big heave, which (I'm still bigger and stronger) I can contain, either resisting it or allowing it to overpower me.

Symbolically, the child can experience this as an opportunity to show how displeased they are at having to follow instructions. If they then overwhelm me, they may feel, 'Now I've shown him!' Because all of this occurs in play, there is no direct challenge to my authority and I don't show myself to be weak; I just acknowledge my child's power.

If I've resisted their attempts to overpower me, they realise, 'He's still bigger than me and I have to give in to him.' If I appear more powerful, it doesn't diminish their power, just underlines that the balance still lies with me, the parent. Importantly, my symbolic 'victory' can be tempered with my observations about how strong my child is and how much effort they put in. I can be magnanimous in my 'win' so that it doesn't belittle my child but lets them know that ultimately I can manage them.

Play like this adds security and trust to my relationship with my children because they consistently learn where they stand with me. I become consistent and predictable to them because we play the game to the same rules and in the same safe space.

Toileting: a landmark moment in gaining responsibility

Toilet-training is a big deal for toddlers and their parents. It's a key time in family life when children begin to take responsibility for themselves and their behaviour. We want them to grow into their responsibility and we want them to feel secure in their ability to regulate certain behaviours, such as weeing and pooing. We need to remember that it's a significant developmental progression for our children that should leave them feeling good about themselves.

We often underestimate the importance of these shifts for children. We may be tempted to look at toilet-training as a chore, an unwelcome task, rather than as the opportunity it is to increase our child's independence and responsibility. When the process doesn't go smoothly we can see the knock-on effect in terms of the child's confidence or their sense of themselves as able. Difficulty in mastering bowel or bladder function can dent a child's self-esteem.

Resisting the pressure to toilet-train too soon

Endless nappy-changing or the pressure to have children trained in time to start pre-school may mean we push our children onto the potty with undue haste. All the collected wisdom about toilet-training suggests that if we begin too soon, and our children aren't ready, the process takes longer and everyone (the child included) ends up frustrated. In such cases, if training has been forced and stressful, we usually find that our toddler shows anxiety about letting go (literally and psychologically) of their babyhood.

The signs that your child is ready to toilet-train

Happily, children will show signs of their readiness to take responsibility for using the toilet. The signs of readiness to look out for are:

* Showing interest in the toileting habits of others

* Asking to use the toilet or potty

* Warning us in advance of their intention to do a wee or a poo

* Having regular and predictable bowel movements

* Showing interest in being independent generally.

When several of these indicators occur together, we are more likely to be successful. Generally, we begin to see these signs between two and a half and three years of age, although girls may be ready sooner while some boys hit three and a half before they show any indication of it.

Maximising the potential for successful toilet-training

It's worthwhile doing a bit of preparation before you launch into the training. Talk to your toddler and maybe read them some story-books about toilet-training so they know what is about to happen. Buy plenty of pairs of pants, letting your son or daughter choose them. Then decide between either a potty or an insert for the toilet seat.

Once we have explained to our child about using the toilet, the core principle is to reinforce any success and ignore accidents – they will occur. We don't necessarily need a star chart: simple praise is often enough, although star charts are public acknowledgement of our child's achievements. If there has been an accident, it may be a good idea to bring a child to the toilet as soon as we notice and suggest they 'finish off' there.

Toddlers are not the best judges of urgency, as regards their need to use the loo. If they say they need to go, you can be pretty sure that the deluge is imminent. Be as quick as you can in getting them to the loo with their pants down in time. Don't be shy about letting them squirt against a wall, into a drain or behind a bush if you get caught outdoors.

It's always worthwhile carrying several spare pairs of pants – and have plenty of patience! That's the real key to toilet-training. Some children get the hang of it quite quickly; others need lots of reminding and encouraging, but if we hang in there, every child will step up to taking responsibility for their wees and poos.

Potential hitches on the road to being fully trained

Parents tend to hold on to responsibility for tasks that should be managed by their children, and this is a regular feature of persistent toileting problems. Often the root of the difficulty was planted in the early days of training. For example, if parents are over-eager and continue to prompt their child to use the toilet long after they need to, he or she may learn not to bother going to the toilet because their parents will remind them. Sometimes using the toilet is associated with pain, perhaps during a bout of constipation, so a child may become anxious about it. If parents are punitive in response to accidents, children may associate toileting with fear.

Problems with toileting can persist for years, and the tension that builds around constant soiling or wetting can lead to conflict between children and their parents. If children don't toilet-train successfully in their toddler or pre-school years, a negative cycle of interaction may result. Resolving the problem may take more than starting from scratch. Far from toileting being a positive experience, it may become a challenge to family harmony.

A case in point …

Janet's seven-year-old daughter Robin soiled constantly, usually once a day, occasionally twice a day, at worst up to five or six times. Janet had attempted various solutions but nothing had worked. It seemed to her that Robin had difficulty in responding to the signals that her poo was coming so when she could be persuaded to get to a toilet it was too late.

Robin hated her mother telling her to go to the toilet and was angry and resistant to any attempt to talk about it or to solve the immediate problems it caused (having to change her clothes and wash her bum). Janet found she spent most of her time with Robin trying to tune into her physical movements. If she spotted Robin squirming on her chair, she would assume she was trying to hold back a poo and immediately prompted her to go to the toilet. Robin regularly refused, crossly telling her mum she didn't need to go, but sooner or later the smell gave away the truth. Tension was high in the house.

When Robin, Janet and I explored how this had started it became clear that Robin had never been taught mastery of her poos (known as primary encopresis). Janet recalled her crying the first time she had been put on the potty because the poo wouldn't come. Janet was then worried about an apparent blockage. She had become very vigilant about Robin's signs that she needed to go and had her hopping on and off the potty to make sure she caught the poo when it eventually came. From then on 'catching the poo' became a big deal.

Robin looked perplexed as her mum recounted this to me. She had no memory of it. She asked her mum, 'Is that why you still tell me to go all the time?' Janet nodded. Robin then admitted that she sometimes refused to go because her mum was hassling her about it. 'You never let me do anything by myself,' she added. She hated her mum being so overpowering and insistent. Also, she never had to pay heed to her need to go to the loo because it was only a matter of time before her mum told her to.

I explained that Robin's soiling was being reinforced by how 'tuned in' Janet was – it was almost as if she was more aware of Robin's poo than Robin was – and that she had taken a lot of the responsibility for her toileting. For example, she reminded Robin to go, focusing on and aware of Robin's poo rhythms, cleaning her and worrying about her social standing.

I wanted Robin to realise that being in charge of her poo was her responsibility. My aim was to remove Janet from the process. The first step was to get Robin to go to the toilet independently of Janet. That meant she had to take responsibility for going three or four times a day, irrespective of her need, to get her into the habit of sitting on the loo without prompting. Importantly, the gain for Robin was that in showing greater responsibility for her toileting she would be allowed greater responsibility for other aspects of her life, like playing unsupervised within the grounds of their estate.

If accidents still happened, I insisted that Janet respond warmly: 'All right, now you need to go and get yourself clean.' If Robin asked for help, Janet was to decline nicely, reminding Robin that she was big enough to sort it out for herself.

The change in a very short time was dramatic. Robin proved she could sort herself out and, in fact, seemed to relish the opportunity to prove to her mum that she could be responsible. Janet took on board the concept that we need to give children responsibility if we want them to be responsible and allowed Robin greater independence generally (within certain sensible boundaries). Robin's greater sense of freedom, thanks to her mum letting go a bit, reinforced her determination to prove that she could manage, and the soiling stopped.

Some facts about bedwetting

The delay between being trained by day and by night is often frustrating but completely normal. Most children will be dry at night between three and six months after day-time toileting is established. Almost half of all children will wet the bed up to the age of three. Night-time accidents are normal up to the age of seven, with approximately one in ten children still wetting.

Bedwetting appears to be most strongly associated with physiological immaturity. Most children who wet the bed can't help it. There also seems to be a strong genetic or family component: about three-quarters of children whose parents both wet the bed as youngsters will do the same.

Staying dry at night

Staying dry at night depends on how deeply children sleep. Sometimes they may not receive the message from their bladder that it needs to be emptied. Some children develop the capacity to hold wee, and stay dry even if they don't wake. Other children need to be alerted by getting the 'I'm bursting' sensation strongly enough to wake them so they can go to the toilet. Others will get the signal but won't respond to it because it doesn't override their sleep.

It can be helpful to allow children to feel the 'bursting' sensation during the day by getting them to hold on to the wee for a minute or two longer, once they know they need to go. This gives their brain a stronger chance to experience and be aware of what the feeling is telling them. Then, during the night, they may be more conscious of it and wake.

It is worth restricting drinks in the evening to give children a better chance of staying dry. Liquid will, inevitably, be digested and most of it ends up as wee. If it has gone in, it must come out. For the same reason we should always insist on a final visit to the bathroom before our children jump into bed. Night-time nappies, training pants or pull-ups may affect their motivation to try to stay dry. Sometimes simply putting a child to bed without a nappy can kick-start their night-time control: if they don't need to be responsible for getting to the toilet, why would they bother to try?

There are conflicting views on 'lifting' children, the practice of carrying them, usually in their sleep, and sitting them on the loo, typically last thing before we go to bed ourselves. Some believe it can set up bad habits. However, if a child tends to wet the bed, I believe lifting is a good idea. It's true that a child may, consciously or not, come to rely on being lifted so they will be longer in learning to wake themselves or hold on. Deciding whether or not to lift a child last thing at night often comes down to practicalities: it's either that or the hassle of changing sheets and pyjamas – not to mention the distress and sense of failure that bedwetting can set up in a young child. Sometimes only patience and positive thinking are required; control will eventually come.

Discipline that builds children's confidence

Families thrive when children are well disciplined. Our understanding of the term 'discipline', though, is crucial to how effectively we discipline our children. For some people, discipline involves lots of rules and limits, with relentless enforcement, using consequences and punishment for any transgression. This kind of rigid firmness will probably create obedience but also unhappiness and resentment.

I much prefer a style of discipline that has a positive focus and intention. Our job is to guide our children and regulate their behaviour until they are old enough to do this for themselves. I prefer to do this by showing children how we want them to behave, rather than punishing them for the ways in which we don't want them to behave.

Most children are exploring their world and in the process they often make mistakes and create mess. Their exploration can be in opposition to what we are trying to achieve. This is not a reason to punish them. It is a reason to offer them some discipline to guide them so that they make fewer mistakes in the future, create less mess and learn to make better choices.

For many parents, discipline has a negative connotation because it has been associated with punishment or a harsh regimen. This is unfortunate because children need discipline, even if they don't need punishment.

Understanding how punishment operates

Punishment for wrongdoing is a deeply embedded behavioural principle in many families and society at large. It is based on the understanding that when our behaviour leads to negative consequences we are less likely to repeat it. This is a well-researched principle, and it has been effectively proven that when we carry out an action and something bad happens as a direct consequence, we are less inclined to carry out the action again for fear of the consequence. For example, if you touch a hot stove you may burn your finger. When you have been burned, you are unlikely to touch the stove intentionally again.

However, we can be a long time waiting for the world to provide negative consequences to children's (and indeed adults') behaviour, so we have taken the principle and extended it to creating negative consequences where no natural ones exist. Many parents (and parenting educators) like to use the term 'setting consequences' for children because it sounds better than 'setting punishments'. But let's not get too hung up on terminology because, in real terms, created negative consequences are punishments.

For example, there is no naturally occurring negative consequence for taking someone else's money so we create a punishment. If a child takes money from a parent's wallet, they may be grounded, or some other significant privilege is curtailed. If an adult is caught entering a house and taking money, they may be imprisoned.

The severity of a punishment is usually determined by the misbehaviour – the 'punishment fitting the crime'. In theory, a punishment is intended as a deterrent, either as a warning of what might happen if we misbehave or a reminder not to misbehave again for fear of receiving the same punishment. So, according to that logic, the greater or more extreme the misbehaviour, the greater or more extreme the punishment must also be. In practice, most punishment is not just a deterrent; it is also used as a means of retaliation, rather than simple behaviour management. Some punishments are far more extreme than the misbehaviour warrants.

The problems with punishment

For punishments to be effective with young children, they must occur immediately after the misbehaviour and should be clearly associated with it so that the child can learn that the misbehaviour led to the punishment and that not repeating the misbehaviour will avoid repetition of the punishment.

Practically, however, in families, we often achieve neither timely nor appropriate punishment. Sometimes we use punishments that are not linked to the misbehaviour (such as sending a child to a 'naughty step' for everything they do wrong). In this case the punishment won't seem like a natural consequence for the misbehaviour and a child may not realise what behaviour they are expected to change.

Sometimes we delay the imposition of a punishment for so long that a child fails to associate it with the original misbehaviour. For instance, if we tell a child on Monday that they won't get their pocket money on Friday because they hit their sister, by Friday nobody may remember why the pocket money was stopped.

Sometimes the same kind of misbehaviour elicits different punishments, depending on which parent is there or what kind of mood the parent is in: a child who spits out his food may be sent away from the table by one parent or slapped by the other. The child may simply learn not to spit in front of one parent rather than learning not to spit at all.

A final issue arises when we put a punishment in place, then can't, won't or don't implement it, perhaps because we realise later that it is too severe, or too difficult to carry out, or we simply forget (letting a child out to play two weeks into a month-long grounding). In such situations we show ourselves to be inconsistent and unwilling or unable to stick to our word.

Practically, then, punishments can confuse children because they may not get a clear, consistent message about their behaviour when it prompts different responses, depending on changing variables.

The emotional impact of punishment

When we punish children it has a significant emotional impact on them. Typically, the kind of scenarios considered in some research conducted in the US were parents' responses to their toddlers' temper tantrums. The most problematic were parents' dismissal of their behaviour ('Don't be silly – stop acting like a baby'), and sending the child to their room. One of the researchers wrote, 'When parents punish their toddlers for becoming angry or scared, children learn to hide their emotions instead of showing them. These children may become increasingly anxious when they have these feelings because they know they'll face negative consequences.'

Unfortunately, many parenting educators promote the use of 'consequences' to discourage children from negative or bold behaviour, almost to the exclusion of any other form of discipline. This is an unbalanced approach to rearing our children. Even if the behaviourist theory that underpins the use of 'consequences' is sound, it cannot be the only way we try to regulate children's behaviour.

On the surface a child's behaviour may change after punishment, and pure behaviourist theory says that this is all that counts. However, even though behaviourists may not like to acknowledge it, we all, including children, have an emotional world, which interacts with our behaviour and influences it. We must, therefore, consider the negative emotional impact of the punishments we mete out and balance it with the positive emotional impact of rewarding positive behaviour.

A case in point ...

Judy was mum to two pre-schoolers, Emma, aged just three, and Jemima, two. There were eleven months between the girls. Judy's dilemma was how she could discipline them, especially Jemima, who had a 'very demanding personality'. She described how Jemima threw tantrums when she was disciplined. Judy was upset by how much the girls fought with each other and often felt helpless to intervene or improve the atmosphere in the house. She felt she was constantly giving out to them and the house felt like a battleground most of the time.

Judy explained that she constantly had to threaten and punish them before they listened to her, and that neither of the girls seemed to respect her. She was quick to tell me of how she tried not to 'let them away with anything'. Punishments included sending them to the naughty step, occasionally smacking them (more often Jemima than Emma) and regularly shouting at them.

Judy was in a disheartening position in her family life. She seemed trapped in a negative cycle of interaction with her girls. They got frustrated, they fought; when they fought, she got cross; if she got cross, she punished them; once she had punished them, they became more upset; as they got more upset or frustrated, she ended up punishing them again.

I explained to Judy that most toddlers and pre-schoolers are not malicious. Certainly they throw tantrums, get frustrated and act without thinking, but this is natural in children so young. They needed to learn how they should be acting, not simply be told, or punished for, what they should not do.

There are very few small children who are wilfully bold but many do things we don't like. I wasn't surprised to hear that Judy's children fought constantly because many children of their age have a low tolerance of frustration and may easily react in a physical way. That Judy also threatened and spanked them demonstrated to them an aggressive way of interacting with others. I felt that this, too, influenced them in hitting out at each other.

Judy needed alternatives for dealing with her children. I wanted to encourage her to move away from a punishment-based system of discipline to a system based on using a positive relationship with the children to influence them to behave well. If nothing else, I wanted her to attempt a more positive relationship with them to break the increasingly negative cycle of interaction that she had fallen into with them.

The key to building a positive relationship, which worked for Judy, was to spend more time playing and having fun with them. Like many parents, Judy was busy and had taken opportunities when the girls were quiet, or playing well together, to do household chores. Indeed, it had seemed that she only ever went to the girls when they fought or misbehaved. If they had learned anything from this, it was probably that misbehaving got them attention from their mother.

Once Judy was spending time with them when they were behaving well, she had the opportunity to 'catch them being good', to notice and comment on their good behaviour. By praising them for it she saw more of it, and they learned that they could get as much, if not more, of her attention for being good.

I encouraged Judy to use distraction as a method for diverting them from potential rows or fights. This meant she didn't have to directly address every little issue that arose with them and didn't need to be in conflict with them as much. I also persuaded her to ignore most of the minor tantrums and misbehaviour, further strengthening the girls' unconscious awareness that they had more of a relationship with her when they were well behaved.

Judy really took on board the notion that her girls were essentially good children who occasionally did naughty things. She no longer wanted to label them naughty and dumped the idea of putting them on a 'naughty step' for misbehaviour. She still gave the girls some time apart, on occasion, to let their tempers cool or to prevent minor rows from escalating. Importantly, though, the message the girls now received was that this was a positive option to calm down, rather than a rejecting punishment for being bold.

Judy also found that when she made games out of tasks like tidying, dressing, bathing, and so on, she attracted much less opposition. By making these tasks fun she was more relaxed, which transferred to the girls so that they sensed their mum enjoyed being with them. When they felt loved and positively acknowledged by her, they were naturally more responsive to her requests and less oppositional.

Catching children being good is more effective than punishing them for acting boldly

Judy's experience shows how much the emotional aspect of our relationship with our children impacts on how effectively we can discipline them. By creating positive relationships we can use our connection with them to guide them towards appropriate behaviour without resorting to punishment.

Instead, when we rely on the positive elements of behavioural theory, reinforcing the behaviour we want to see more of, we not only see more good behaviour in evidence but reap positive emotional benefits for our children too. Punishment can lead children to feel angry, upset and resentful; praise will lead them to feel proud, capable and loved. This boosts their self-esteem and increases their sense that they are respected.

Why slapping and time-out don't get positive results

Most parents who have slapped their children will say that they only ever do so as a last resort when they feel frustrated by their children's continued misbehaviour. They will say that they never intend to slap hard; they just want to 'make the point' that a particular behaviour is unacceptable.

In my experience of working with children who have been slapped, they rarely learn that certain behaviour is bold and they must not repeat it. Instead, they pick up much more complicated messages that have far more potentially damaging consequences.

When they are slapped, children see an adult getting angry and hitting out when others don't do as the adult wants. Because children model their behaviour on that of the adults around them, it is likely that a child will learn to hit others (children or adults) who frustrate them or don't do what they want.

Also, a consequence needs to be associated with specific negative behaviour for a child to learn not to carry it out again. In practice, most parents who slap do so towards the end of a long row with, or series of misbehaviour from, their child. The child doesn't know exactly why they have been slapped. In fact, they are more likely to believe they were slapped because their parent was angry than because of any particular misbehaviour.

According to behavioural theory, all consequences lose their effectiveness in time. As slapping loses its effectiveness as a punishment (which it will do), the temptation is to up the ante in terms of the frequency with which a parent slaps or the strength they apply as a means of trying to 'get through' to their child. This can lead to children being seriously hurt and physically abused.

In a similar way, time-out as a consequence for misbehaviour sends all the wrong signals to children and creates the power struggles and disrespect we try to avoid. Most parents who employ punishment time-out use it as a consequence for myriad types of misbehaviour, from hitting to non-compliance and everything in between; their child may not take the correct learning from the consequence and may not grasp what they need to stop doing.

Also, parents who put their child in punishment time-out rarely do so without engaging them in a row or discussion. This is because few children willingly accept time-out (or any punishment) and will try to argue their point. As this discussion or row develops, the parent may end up giving more individual attention to their child. He or she may be unconsciously and unintentionally 'hooked' into interacting with the child. This attention, even though it is negative, can be reinforcing for a child who just wants to be noticed by their parent: they may learn that misbehaving gets them uninterrupted one-to-one time with a parent.

Children quickly learn that naughty children are sent to a 'naughty step'. If they are repeatedly sent there, they may come to believe that they are naughty or bold. This may have damaging consequences for their self-esteem. Once they believe they are bold, what is the point in being good? If they know themselves to be bold, can they ever know themselves to be good?

Effective ways to discipline children

Instead of relying on punishment, I suggest that you try these positive discipline techniques instead.

* **Managing the space**. If a pen is on the floor, it can be picked up and used to write on the wall. If the dishware cupboard is low or unlocked, plates or glasses can be pulled out by curious toddlers and accidentally broken. We need to keep an eye on the environment that our toddlers live in and make sure that their opportunities to cause havoc are limited. The less havoc they cause, the less we need to correct them.

* **Staying close by**. Toddlers create more trouble when they're unsupervised. If we keep close to them, we'll spot potential accidents or tantrums and can often intervene to avoid a problem occurring.

* **Lending a helping hand**. Toddlers get enormously frustrated when they can't do things. We can reduce this by offering enough help to get them over the hump of a problem. For example, if a particular block won't squeeze through the wrong hole, we can reorient the holder so that the block is lined up with the right hole. This might prevent the whole contraption being flung in fury.

* **Distraction**. Toddlers have wonderfully short attention spans and that means that they can be easily distracted from

the source of frustration or difficulty. Suggesting that they help you do the vacuuming could prove just the diversion from a brewing tantrum.

❋ **Planned ignoring**. We don't have to fight every battle with our children. Especially if we feel that they are just attention-seeking and as long as nobody is in line to get hurt, we can often ignore them. As soon as they stop misbehaving, we can shower them with attention.

❋ **Being directive**. Sometimes toddlers just need to be reminded of what they have to do so we need to tell them firmly. Sometimes we need to back it up with physical direction, perhaps bringing them to the bathroom and handing them their toothbrush because 'It's time to brush your teeth!'

❋ **Creating breathing space**. Despite our best intentions and interventions the world is sometimes too much for toddlers and they have tantrums. As long as they're safe and not hurting anyone it's okay to give them some space and time to calm down. We can empathise with their distress or anger, saying something like, 'You seem very upset … When you're feeling calmer we can sort this out and I'll be in the kitchen till then.' This isn't a punishment, just an opportunity to let tempers die down and allow calm to return.

Setting limits

Of course, as part of our discipline for children, we need to structure their world. They need limits and boundaries to keep them safe and stop them creating problems for themselves or others. We use physical boundaries like fences, stair- and garden gates to prevent small children getting into situations where they could get hurt. We use psychological limits and boundaries for the same purpose.

For example, with older children, we ask them to come home at certain times, tell them to go to bed to ensure they get enough rest, insist they wear enough layers to avoid getting cold or restrict their use of media so they aren't overwhelmed by too many competing influences.

It's helpful if we can establish our authority early in our children's lives, when we still have the physical power to limit and put boundaries around them and their behaviour. When they are small we can be directive; we can enforce small consequences and show them we mean what we say. If we establish this early, we will find that our limits are simply not challenged.

If we miss the opportunity to establish this, it's always possible to introduce it later, but we may have to make more effort to teach our children that we mean what we say. We may have to rely on threatening consequences for a time, and it is equally important that we balance this with plenty of praise for positive behaviour. If we are to apply consequences, we must regularly 'catch them being good'. We must also try to ensure that any consequences we use are as natural as possible and are the very minimum required to motivate a child not to repeat the misbehaviour.

Our goal in disciplining our children is to give them some internal sense of discipline and a moral code that will allow them to make wise, safe and good choices through their lives.

We need to show them respect, in our consideration of their needs, views and perspectives, from an early age. Children can be involved in discussions about family rules, limits and even fair consequences. When we include them in this way, they will feel respected and will be more likely to adhere to rules and limits if they have signed up to them. Indeed, they can come to internalise them as values they inherently believe in.

Let's take an example of a four-year-old who wants to go for a walk with you but won't wear their coat. Here is how that conversation may go in many homes.

Parent: Okay, put on your coat now so we can go to the shop.

Child: No!

Parent: Put on your coat or we're not going.

Child: I hate that coat.

Parent: I don't care if you like it or not, you need to wear it because it's cold. Now, put it on or we're not going. I'll count to three.

Child: (Starts crying.)

Parent: One ... two ... (no sign of child putting on coat and so parent says angrily) ... three. Right, that's it, no shop for you. Take off those shoes. You are so bold! Why can't you do the simplest things? It's only a coat, for God's sake.

Child: (Cries harder and starts screaming in frustration at losing the opportunity to go to the shop.)

Parent: (Getting increasingly angry) Stop crying or there'll be no TV this afternoon either. Stop it! Stop it now! I'm warning you ...

This interaction will probably lead to the child losing his TV time later, and both parent and child will likely have a hard day, filled with resentment and bad feeling.

An alternative approach to the same situation, which is more respectful and inclusive of the child's feelings and opinions, may go like this:

Parent: Okay, put on your coat now so we can go to the shop.

Child: No!

Parent: Oh, you sound like you don't want to wear this coat.

Child: I hate that coat.

Parent: Oh, you hate this coat. That's tricky. You need to wear a coat because it's cold outside. What can we do to solve our problem?

Child: Nothing, I'm not wearing that coat.

Parent: Well, you need to wear something warm.

> *Child:*   No, I don't!
>
> *Parent:*   You may not want to wear anything, but I don't want you to get sick because you catch a cold.
>
> *Child:*   (Makes no response.)
>
> *Parent:*   How about I put the coat in the bag and if you get cold you can put it on?
>
> *Child:*   (Shrugs shoulders.)

The most likely outcome here is that the two head off to the shop (with the parent gritting their teeth!). Then, either the child runs to keep warm or accepts the offer of the coat because he realises that it is very cold. Here he experiences the natural consequence of not wearing his coat (getting cold) and is much more likely to learn that he needs to put it on before going out in future. Indeed, the parent can gently draw out this learning by saying something like, 'Wow, it really is cold so it's a good thing you have a nice warm coat to put on. If we wear coats from the time we leave the house we never get so cold.'

The interaction results in the parent getting their way (the child wears the coat) or the parent learns that their child didn't need the coat. Ultimately they discovered the outcome by trial and error rather than relying on the parent's greater knowledge and wisdom (which may not always be infallible). What is important is that the parent respected the opinion of their four-year-old enough to try out the child's preferred option. Depending on the situation, you may not be able to be so flexible, although usually this is only the case if the potential outcome of your child's choice is dangerous for them or others.

Another ending to the scenario above may be:

> *Parent:*   Oh, you hate this coat. That's tricky. You need to wear a coat because it's cold outside. What can we do to solve our problem?
>
> *Child:*   Nothing. I'm not wearing that coat.
>
> *Parent:*   Well, you need to wear something warm.

Child: No, I don't!

Parent: You may not want to wear anything, but I don't want you to get sick because it's freezing outside.

Child: (Makes no response.)

Parent: I'm going to have to put this coat on you anyway, even though you hate it, because getting frostbite is more dangerous than you being upset.

Child: (Struggles, cries and screams.)

Parent: (Holding their child firmly) I can see and hear that you seem really upset at having to wear the coat and I'm sorry you have to do something you don't like. Sometimes we don't get the choices that we want and that is very hard. You may feel less cross in a while.

Child: (Continues to scream and protest for a few minutes up the road until the neighbours' dog runs over and distracts him.)

I'm not advocating a family democracy (not until we're coping with adult children still in our homes anyway) but we need to create a form of benevolent authority in which we listen respectfully to our children, even if we have to make the final decision.

Creating thriving attitudes to food and eating

The attitudes we develop towards food and eating in our childhood can have lasting effects on how we eat throughout our lives. They are most strongly influenced by parents. How we talk about food, react to food or fussy eating, discuss body-weight or -image, or how we treat our bodies in relation to our eating or, perhaps, dieting will have an impact on our children. It is important, therefore, that we pay attention to the influence we bring to bear.

We need to be careful not to associate food or eating with rewards or punishments. Typically, we offer sweet treats as an inducement for either good behaviour or successfully eating dinner. This kind of association can set up lifelong habits in which sweets, chocolate and other food become a reward. If we are given treats to make up for disappointments, they may become a comfort at any time of stress.

Sweets, chocolate and desserts will usually seem like treats to children because they don't get them regularly. It is fine to give them treats occasionally, but the key is not to associate them with particular behaviour or moods. So, if there is to be dessert because it's the weekend, the dessert is associated with the day, not with your child and what they have done.

As with many aspects of parenting, our own actions will speak louder than words when it comes to how our children pick up our attitudes, beliefs and values. When in doubt, if we show positive attitudes and behaviour in relation to food and eating, there is a much higher likelihood that our children will develop similarly positive ideas. A recent study showed that babies and young children are susceptible to the emotions of others to the extent that seeing enjoyment in the faces of adults may trigger the same emotional response in a child. So if we seem to be enjoying certain foods, young children may believe they will like them too.

A child who makes his or her own food choices, within the options offered to them, and is allowed the responsibility to do so will thrive. A family who can allow mealtimes to become social events, in which food can be nurturing and nutritious (rather than the source of conflict and fighting), will also thrive.

Understanding fussy or faddy eating

When we think about it, it makes sense that humans are fussy about food. After all, certain substances are harmful. We rarely mind when other adults express food preferences. Think, for example, of how you respond to a friend telling you they only like hard-boiled eggs, never eat spinach or that they're vegetarian. In each case we're likely to be tolerant and understanding; we assume they have reasons for their choices, and we don't take the responsibility of determining their diet from them.

But we do determine the diets of our children. Phrases like 'Eat your greens', 'You must eat a bit of the chicken' and 'If you don't eat all your dinner, there'll be no dessert for you,' are commonplace at dinner tables around the country.

Attempting to force children to eat particular foods does not encourage them to be responsible eaters. It encourages them to conform, if they feel your power is too great, or to be oppositional if they want to push a different view or opinion. We so badly want our children to thrive physiologically, as well as psychologically and emotionally, but not allowing them to choose what they eat threatens all three opportunities to thrive.

Children can make healthy food choices

Imagine letting your children choose between a few different foods. Imagine letting even small babies handle their food, lick or suck it from their fingers. Imagine letting children determine when they're full. Imagine allowing children more control about what and how much they eat.

Remarkably, when children have free rein to choose from available foods, they tend to find a balance between all the major food groups. They may eat mainly carbohydrate for a time, then mainly protein, but over several weeks their diet is balanced overall. I think it feels too much of a risk for most of us to give them complete freedom, because we worry that they won't eat enough (or the right things) to survive.

It is never too late to start to give them increased responsibility and choice. What we need to remember is that an older child may never have been allowed to choose freely and may not know what to do. Rather than turning over the kitchen to them and telling them to sort themselves out if they don't want to eat what we're offering, we need slowly to increase the number of choices they are given.

'Would you like peas or beans?'; 'Do you want a big spoonful or a little one of the mashed potato?'; 'Do you want more now or will I leave the rest of your dinner in case you're hungry later?' Children will make such choices if they're genuinely free to do so. Being free means that they don't fear negative consequences for either choice and can be confident that we will remain warm and connected with them, no matter what they choose.

The role of control in fussy eating

Allowing your children more responsibility for their own eating is a great antidote to the fussiness we see that is often bound up in a power-and-control dynamic between us and our children. When we insist on certain foods, and certain amounts of food, to be eaten, our children may resist.

In fact, they hold quite a lot of power when it comes to food; refusal to eat is one of the few areas that they are fully in charge of. We can't force them to eat something they don't want. Children realise this so when we try to coerce or cajole them into eating, they can show us just how powerful they are.

The battle is rarely about greens or the piece of chicken. The food is merely the backdrop for a deeper struggle to show who in the family is most powerful. What a shame that our children's potentially healthy attitude to food has to suffer in a power struggle.

A case in point ...

The Matterly family comprised Maura, Peter, James, aged four, and Siobhan, six months. Maura and Peter came to see me because James 'eats nothing'. From when he was weaned, dinner times had been a battle in the Matterly house. Maura described how they had 'tried everything' to get James to eat what they considered to be proper dinners, to no avail.

She told me about the fights she had with James over his refusal to eat 'proper food'. He had regularly sat at the table for hours while his mother refused to let him leave until his plate was cleared. These stand-offs had often led to a screaming match, food thrown into the bin, and James being marched off to bed.

In that first session I carried out a 'food history' with each parent and got them to talk about their memories of food, mealtimes and eating in their own families when they were growing up. Peter had never had any issues with food. He ate a pretty balanced diet. However, a sister had developed anorexia aged fourteen when he was just seven. He recalled the tensions and the fighting at their family dinner table as his sister became thinner and thinner and eventually refused to sit with the family for meals. He remembered his mother's anguish and anger, and vividly recalled his sister's expressed hatred of his parents. He took his lead from his dad, who had never got involved, just kept his head down.

Maura had grown up in a large family and her mother's main dinner offering was stew, with the same basic taste and watery consistency. Mealtimes were haphazard, with brothers and sisters coming and going, a lot of noise and bustle. She remembered her mother checking that every child ate something; she had insisted on seeing the cleared plate before she let them leave the kitchen. Mealtimes were a pretty joyless affair and eating, Maura felt, was not for pleasure but survival. She didn't remember much chat around the table.

When I enquired about their current food experiences, I discovered that, unsurprisingly, mealtimes in their house were also pretty joyless affairs, with equal amounts of stress and solitude, each person eating their dinner in a perfunctory fashion before leaving the table and separating to different parts of the house. Maura hated cooking and resented having to prepare not just one evening meal but, sometimes, two or three options, depending on James's mood.

The most significant factor, uniting their early food experiences, seemed to me to be the negative attitudes to food that had developed, for different reasons, in their respective family homes.

Maura had clung to the belief that eating everything you were given was the most important facet of a meal. Anxiety about failing in her duty as a mother if her children didn't eat everything was a daily pressure for her. Meanwhile Peter had learned to eat and otherwise keep his mouth shut to avoid drawing anger or stress his way. This grim and somewhat soulless dynamic had pervaded their current family food experiences with James.

Addressing the parents' stresses, anxieties and withdrawal from food caused a big shift in the family's eating habits. Peter and Maura each did a cookery course, and I encouraged them to share the responsibility for cooking. I asked them to give James a break from the pressure to eat what they cooked and, rather, to ensure that he just joined them for each meal. At the meal I insisted that all talk veer away from what and how much was being eaten and that instead it focused on each person in turn, what they were up to and how their day had been. I gave Peter and Maura a list of topics they might chat about at dinner to help them get into a new habit of social rather than functional eating.

Although it took time, the tension at the table reduced. They both commented that James seemed to notice and appreciate his dad's involvement in cooking and mealtimes. Although James still didn't eat a wide variety of foods, neither parent seemed unhappy. Instead, they felt that the stress of mealtimes was so reduced that they all enjoyed their food more. Maura, particularly, felt freed from her previous beliefs that getting her children to eat was the only way to be a good mother. Weaning Siobhan was proving much more relaxed than it had been with James. In fact, both parents felt much more competent as parents than they ever had before.

Having a healthy body image

The attitudes we have and the comments we make about how we look and feel about our bodies can affect our children's and teenagers' views of theirs. Invariably we make those comments from when our children are toddlers. If, for example, we constantly say, 'I'm fat,' or complain that we don't exercise enough, or go on a series of diets, we give off clear messages of discomfort or unhappiness with our bodies.

It is far better for us to focus on our health rather than our weight. If we aim for a healthy lifestyle, our eating habits will fall into line with it. Similarly, if we have to talk about our children's eating habits we should always focus on, and emphasise, their health rather than their weight. This way they get the ideal message that their bodies are healthy and strong and that we love them for who they are and not how they look.

Food and eating as part of a healthy lifestyle

We need to create a situation in which food is only part of the maintenance of a healthy lifestyle for our family; we must also build other things, like exercise, into our family life. We might include taking regular walks, or perhaps going swimming together. We want to make exercise a fun, rewarding and regular activity rather than a means to an end.

Other ways to bring about healthy attitudes to food and eating include involving our children in the preparation of nutritious meals, letting them know that it's okay to eat when they're hungry and to refuse food when they're not. Children thrive, physically and emotionally, when we create the right atmosphere about food and nutrition.

Making time and space for family meals that nurture and connect

In the right emotional atmosphere, children and families thrive, much as plants do better with a good balance of sun, water and nutrients from the soil. A kind, nurturing family environment is an essential part of that nourishing emotional climate. Regular family mealtimes offer a chance to create it. The best time to develop the habit of family meals is during the toddler and pre-school years.

Benefits of family meals

Research supports the notion that family mealtimes allow children to thrive. Those who sit with their family for regular meals are less likely to smoke, take drugs and drink alcohol. They tend to do better in school, have fewer mental-health problems, and eat a more balanced and healthy diet.

When we eat together, we can learn from each other, through conversation, about the values, morals and beliefs we each hold. We increase our opportunities to bond and form relationships with our children, which boosts their sense of security, confidence and self-esteem.

We are pulled in many directions on a daily basis. Frequently it can seem that there isn't enough time to get everything done. Family mealtimes can easily become a casualty of our busy lifestyles, which is a pity because mealtimes may be the best and only time when everyone in the family can gather.

As your children grow older, it is important for them that there are times in the day when they have a chance to talk to parents rather than simply passing them in a whirl of activity. If we don't develop the habit of set times for catching up and sharing food during the toddler years, we may find that our family feels fractured. If our children are older, family meals may be the perfect way to reconnect.

A case in point ...

The Smyth family comprised Shauna, Jack and their three children, Melissa, aged twelve, Samuel, nine, and Julia, seven. Shauna and Jack came to me about the level of fighting between the children. There was a constant heightened tension in the house, with a pervading undercurrent of hostility that threatened to erupt. Things had been manageable up to about three years ago, although they felt there had always been rivalry between the children, whether it was about who sat next to which parent when they went out to dinner, or who decided what to watch on TV.

Shauna ran a successful interior-design consultancy. Jack had been promoted at work the previous year, increasing his stress and his working hours with his salary. They frequently depended on their au pair to do everything from cook for the children, to cleaning and the family laundry. She also looked after the children until late every evening when one or other parent got home or returned with whichever child had been at one of their multitude of extra-curricular activities.

As I probed more, there seemed to be almost no time when the five of them were all together. They had tried, they explained, to go out to dinner on Friday nights but recently it had become tiresome and embarrassing because of the children's squabbles; they had dropped it in favour of getting a take-out, which they rarely ate together because the children disappeared to the TV room with their plates.

As I listened to Shauna and Jack I felt strongly that the children seemed an inconvenience to them, notwithstanding that their having come to see me suggested they must care about their family life. I put this to them, expecting neither of them to accept my observation. Remarkably, though, they looked at each other and Jack admitted they had both reached the point at which they wondered why they had had children. It was this that had prompted them to meet me. They felt their family was slipping away and they wanted to rescue it.

Shauna's own parents, I discovered, had separated when she was twelve. Before that they had led increasingly separate lives; each parent had been successful in their own right. I think Shauna saw this as the 'writing on the wall' in her relationship with Jack. She feared that the stress of home life combined with their heavy work schedules was creating a tension between them that threatened the whole family's disintegration.

The key to healing any cracks in this family was that its members should spend more positive time together. It seemed that neither parent was properly available to the children. They were overworked, stressed and snappy. The children had been cared for by a succession of inexperienced au pairs and it was no wonder they were badly behaved. At their ages, they still needed a lot of parental time, attention and behavioural guidance. It was unfair to expect an au pair to provide this. Many family interactions had become negative and no one was focused on helping parents and children to connect and thrive.

I built family meals into the centre of the family's rejuvenation. I wanted the children to see their parents frequently to allow them to rekindle their relationships with them and each other. I felt that a good proportion of the children's fighting was over the limited attention available to them from either parent. Increasing their parents' availability, would, I felt, help the children to realise that they didn't need to fight to be noticed.

Getting home at a reasonable time so that the family could eat together was a huge commitment for Shauna and Jack to make and involved a major rethink of their priorities. That they invested in this and achieved it sent a powerful message to their children. Their presence and the interest they showed in the emotional life of their children's schools, friendships and activities showed the children that they were important and valued. Creating a space for a family mealtime was the single most successful intervention for this family as it rekindled a togetherness that had been lost in the busyness of their lives.

Shauna and Jack also had to do a certain amount of limit-setting and showing themselves to be back in charge, but even this was easier to achieve when the opportunity for building relationships was increased.

Tips for making family meals into social occasions

Increasing the social aspect of meals means including everybody, by scheduling a meal at a time when we are all at home. This may not work every day, given how busy we can be, but just one family meal a week can make a difference. When our children are very young, we should pull them close to the table in high-chairs so they are part of the group rather than sitting outside it, and get booster seats so that toddlers can sit equally with older children or adults.

Beforehand we may like to think up some topics to talk about – the activities of the day, plans for later the next day, what happened at play-times, school, friends, teachers, uncles, aunts, things from our own childhoods, stories from when our children were younger, and so on.

Involving children in the preparation of the meal and the setting of the table connects them to the occasion. Even toddlers can help with mashing or stirring. They feel some ownership of the meal when they have been involved in its creation.

Family meals can be a source of fun and, irrespective of the food that is eaten, a very nurturing part of a family's day. When we determine what to prioritise among the many competing demands of family life, let's think about mealtimes, the warmth, nurturing and togetherness that comes from eating together.

Establishing family traditions to cherish

Akin to family mealtimes, the development of family traditions is another opportunity to create a warm and nurturing environment for our families to thrive in. Traditions frequently evolve in our children's toddler years since this may be the first time we make Christmas a big deal, or that they are conscious of what we may do for them on their birthday. Even weekly routines can become traditional, or at least habitual, if children invest emotional energy in them.

We know that certain activities or experiences earn the 'tradition' moniker when they 'have' to be done. When we hear the clamour of eager children or see their expressions of disappointment, we know we're on to a good thing.

Benefits of traditions and habits

Traditions are a little rock – a bit of stability or consistency – that can anchor families in otherwise stormy times. They don't have to cost. In my opinion the best traditions are those that will be remembered with warmth, affection and appreciation. They strengthen the relationships within our family. Shared experiences are a point of contact between family members exclusive to them; they offer a sense of community and togetherness. Traditions that are passed down to us provide continuity through the generations and connect us to the strength of our extended families. Traditions nurture the soul because they instil goodwill.

Whether habit or tradition, they are valued by children and adults alike

More often we consider annual events that follow a predictable routine or structure to be 'traditional'. When something happens more frequently we may downgrade it to a family habit (for example, 'Friday night is family movie night'). Even habits are important (as long as they are positive) because they offer children the consistency and predictability that will help to reduce anxiety or relieve stress. Most family habits are focused around being together and enjoying a shared activity or spending some special time with the children.

Positive habits of thriving families

* Nightly, or regular, storytime with children of all ages. (There is something about a spoken story that fires the imagination and builds closeness between speaker and listener.)

❋ Weekly family movie night. (It's hard to beat the moment of cuddliness as everyone snuggles up to zone-out for a while.)

❋ At least one meal a week that everyone loves and can look forward to eating together. (Homemade pizza night is the winner in my house.)

❋ Regular family walks, or some other exercise we can all do together (no matter the weather!).

❋ Regular family meetings (see Chapter 4).

❋ Rotate children's photos and drawings on the fridge so that no one feels left out.

❋ Volunteer together (when children are older) to help people less fortunate or able than your family. (It can help us all to appreciate the good in our own family.)

❋ Try to make a regular plan to spend time with each individual child. (Children need our undivided personal attention.)

Some great Christmas or birthday traditions to try

I have included some suggestions here, but the kinds of annual traditions you can create are limited only by your imagination.

❋ Stirring the Christmas and birthday cake mix allows for two wishes each year!

❋ Keep themed story books, carol CDs or movie DVDs just for Christmas time.

❋ An advent calendar counts down the days to Christmas, building the excitement before the day.

❋ Attend a charity carol service.

❋ Decorate the house with your children before Christmas or a birthday.

❋ Hope Santa might leave the same gift in a stocking each year.

❋ Leaving the same kind of snack for Santa and Rudolph provides similar continuity.

❁ Make or buy a new tree decoration for each child every year, and remember to date them.

❁ Do an activity on Christmas Day (like a walk) and take a moment to remember those who are not with your family any more.

❁ Create a tradition for opening presents (take turns, or roll a die and get a six to be able to open a gift; wait until each gift is savoured before moving to another).

❁ Have a family sleep-over in your bedroom on the night before a birthday to mark the day as special.

❁ Try to have a least one party game or food that appears every year.

❁ Take a birthday photo and measure your child's height on the wall or doorframe; it builds to an amazing record of growth and maturity.

04

THRIVING AT HOME AND AT SCHOOL

Starting school and the primary years: a big step for all the family

When children start primary school, many of us breathe a sigh of relief. Entry to 'big school' marks another transition in our developmental journey as a family. The years that follow, until children reach the age of about twelve, can seem the most settled, emotionally and psychologically. It is often a period in which many families can consolidate, draw breath and think about what they are doing. The novelty and flurry of baby- and toddlerhood can give way to a more thoughtful, considered approach. We may even feel we know what we're doing!

However, our children are increasing their independence and doing more outside the family. There is a greater, or at least a different, draw on our parental time and attention. As their interests and activities expand, we can feel pushed to keep up with them. We may be delighted that they are trying new sports or pastimes but we have to invest heavily in getting them there and often staying while they do their thing.

On top of that, some parents return to work outside the home, or those parents already at work may increase their hours or take on greater responsibility; childcare issues may have been resolved now that the children are at school. So, while we may feel more competent or knowledgeable as a parent, we may also continue to

'Why? But why?' The inquisitive mind

Children ask many questions. They are exploring their world and trying to fit new knowledge into the understanding they already have. We all have schemas, or set ways, in which we think about things; when we acquire new information we have to either fit it into the schema we already have or change the schema to accommodate it.

This is complicated yet we all do it, unconsciously at times. Children are no different, but they tend to be more obvious in their consideration; new information leads to further questioning, often to a series of 'But why ...?'

feel driven to distraction by the busy nature of family life, as we are increasingly drawn in different directions. It is easy for 'family' to get lost in the competing needs of individual members and for thriving to be replaced by hanging on.

Reason and the older child

The ability to talk to children, knowing they understand and will respond, changes how we can deal with them and their behaviour. We no longer have the same dependence on simple behavioural principles because we can reason and rationalise with them. When we encounter problems we can talk them through and children can learn to solve them. This is an opportunity for children to develop skills in critical thinking and reasoning.

Naturally, that means we must allow children to be part of the problem-solving process. Many of us cling to the power and responsibility that comes with having made all the decisions. Even though children in primary school like to grapple with abstract concepts like rules, honesty, justice and fairness, we can sometimes queries, often in rapid succession. In theory, this is great as it reflects real growth. In practice, it can be wearing.

During a protracted 'But why . . .?' session, it is easy to become snappy or disengaged. We lose enthusiasm for the topic, feel bamboozled by its increasing complexity, inadequate with regard to our own knowledge and tormented or distracted by the endless questions in the midst of the other twenty jobs we may have to finish. It may be a challenge to put on a smile and keep answering. That's why it's good to know that the 'stream of consciousness' questioning is part of a thriving development.

exclude them from decision-making because we continue to know best. We sometimes forget that children are clever and capable, and treat them as if they were younger and less able.

The changing emotional landscape

As children get older, they become increasingly self-conscious in relation to and in comparison with other children and adults. They will think about their and others' appearance and may even define themselves by how they look, what they do, their clothes or possessions.

Usually they demonstrate self-consciousness in modesty about their bodies. It is natural for children to become more private long before their teenage years. Children as young as seven may want privacy but, as with many other aspects of childhood, there are no hard and fast rules about the age at which they will express it. It still catches parents by surprise when a child loses his or her previously carefree attitude to their body, or other people's. It may have been driven by parental attitudes and behaviours, but sometimes it comes entirely from a child's sense of him- or herself.

'But *how* do babies get there, Mum?'

Children focus most intensely on same-gender friendships through the primary-school years. In terms of their sexual development, these years are often referred to as the latency period because their sexuality is often hidden and may seem secondary to other areas of their development. Generally, there is very little physical sexual development before the age of ten. Some girls come into puberty between the ages of nine and twelve, with boys tending to reach it later. But irrespective of physical development, psychologically boys and girls continue to develop sexually and will be intrigued by some of the mechanics of sex. When they ask about it, it is best to be truthful, even if we simplify what we tell them.

Don't be afraid to use terms like 'penis', 'vagina', 'sperm' and 'eggs' even with young children. If they don't have a context within which to make sense of the information you give them, it tends to go over their heads anyway. Most children have their own limit for sex-related discussions and may tell you to stop if they don't want to know more! A six-year-old might be happy with the explanation that the daddy's seed joins up with the mummy's seed in her tummy and the baby grows there, but a ten-year-old might ask how the dad's seed gets in to meet the mummy's. This is the time to explain about penises, erections, vaginas and wombs. If you try to describe sperm ejaculation, though, you may be told, 'Enough!' When discussing sex we can always be guided by our children's reaction (their continued interest, inquisitiveness or comparative disinterest), which will indicate how much and how explicitly to tell.

These are also the years in which many children develop fears. They may be rational, an understandable response to traumatic or frightening events, but more often they are irrational. Typical fears of the dark or death, for example, may have no basis in a child's reality, but they worry also about failure, rejection, harm and danger. It is more important that we try to understand and acknowledge their fears than simply try to reassure them. Indeed, unless they believe that you understand how they feel, they are unlikely to accept your reassurance. So, empathise first and reassure afterwards.

The benefits of constructive feedback

The judgements that adults, especially parents, make about children's behaviour and performance are meaningful, and children tend to take them to heart. A nine-year-old girl who considers herself to be good at art may be devastated if she receives negative feedback about a picture she's drawn. Now that they pay more attention to themselves and are beginning to form an identity, perhaps defined by what they are good at, or enjoy, children become attuned to how others perceive them and their abilities. It is all the more important that we are constructive in our feedback.

That is not to say we must be exclusively positive, but it does help! Sometimes it's best to adopt the adage that 'If you can't say anything positive, don't say anything at all.' The judgements we make will influence our children's self-judgements and form an essential backdrop to their developing self-esteem. If we praise their behaviour or performance, they will form positive associations, but as they know us so well, they are likely to spot when we are less than truthful.

So, it is not helpful to lie to them that something is good if it isn't. Instead we can comment positively about the effort they put in, even if the outcome isn't exactly what they wanted. Or we can ask what they think of their own performance or behaviour before we comment. This will give us an idea of their own view. Then, we can constructively identify things that could be done differently or better, if need be, in the context of the hard work that has already been put in.

Imagine that your eleven-year-old son has offered to clean your car. When he shows it to you after he has 'finished', you see that he has missed bits. You could say to him, 'What about all the dirty bits? That car isn't clean yet!' which will probably leave him deflated about his efforts. Or you could say, 'Wow, you've been working really hard. Are you all done? It isn't easy to clean a whole car. Look, even with all of your work there are still some bits waiting to be cleaned. Do you want to do them now or will you have a break before you finish it off?'

Building self-esteem and resilience

High self-esteem lies at the heart of a thriving family. Self-esteem is the judgement we make about how worthy or valuable we feel. I believe that we make two judgements about ourselves that determine the level of our self-esteem: how lovable we are and how capable we are. If we feel neither lovable nor capable, our self-esteem will be low.

We take a lead from the judgements of others in deciding how we should feel about ourselves. Other people, parents especially, have an enormous influence on us and we pay great heed to them and how they treat us. If we feel criticised, dismissed, blamed or somehow unacceptable, we come to believe that these negative attributions are the result of fundamental faults in us. Whether it is parents or siblings who tell a child they are useless, stupid, lazy, ugly, fat, annoying, bold or spoiled, or teachers and peers at school who put them down, children come to believe the negative stuff.

Many of us carry long-standing self-esteem issues from just such comments that were passed about us by our own parents, teachers, brothers, sisters or peers. The more often we heard the criticism, the more we believed it. Once these negatives become core beliefs they are resistant to change or correction. For example, many adults who suffered with dyslexia and struggled to read were labelled as stupid, even though they had average or above average intelligence. As they will tell you, that crippled their self-esteem for years.

Making what we say and do empower our children

We underestimate the power of what we say and do to and with our children even though we know they rely on us to find out about the world and how to make sense of it. Perhaps we don't realise quite how attuned they are to us and our mood, but if we watch them we'll notice that when we're grumpy, the whole house seems on edge and our children are especially badly behaved. In contrast, when we're on top of our game, calm and authoritative with them, they are more amenable and good-humoured.

So, when we explicitly make comments to and about our children, they hear and heed them. On the face of it, they may reject our criticism but internally they will be affected by it. This is one reason I believe that a 'naughty step' can be so counterproductive. If children are regularly sent there, they may grow up still believing they are naughty (only naughty children end up on a naughty step).

We need to take care with comments or criticisms we make because, even if they are said in jest, our children may interpret them as a negative truth about themselves. This will become part of their self-judgement about their value, lovability or capability. It helps to be alert to our own self-esteem in this regard because we may pass on the negative view, based on our own beliefs, that we are not worth much or are not valued. It's hard to value your children if you don't value yourself.

Why self-esteem matters

Research backs up the need to promote children's self-esteem. Children with high self-esteem are more emotionally mature, stable, and have a fair view of themselves that may incorporate positives and some negatives. They have a high frustration tolerance and are more resilient in response to life's ups and downs. In other words, we tend to cope better in the world when our self-esteem is high. The research shows that children with low self-esteem are much more likely to be dependent, conforming and susceptible to peer pressure. If we don't believe in ourselves we are much more likely to follow the crowd than to lead it.

A case in point ...

Cara was a twelve-year-old who came to me as an emergency referral by her GP. She had tried to kill herself by taking a potentially lethal overdose of paracetamol. In the hospital, evidence of self-harming was also discovered in the form of scratches on her wrists, in various stages of healing.

Cara's mum was married to her step-dad, whom her mum had met when Cara was three and married four years later. Cara had a younger half-sister, who was now almost three, and her mum was pregnant again. Cara's biological dad had left when she was only a few months old and she had had no contact with him since. Her mother had told her about her current pregnancy two days before the overdose.

I had spoken with the child and an adolescent psychiatrist who had met her and her mum at the hospital. She remained under the psychiatrist's care although everyone agreed that she would attend me for therapy. The psychiatrist had noted that Cara was very withdrawn and that her mum, Linda, was angry with her for what she had done, now that the initial shock had worn off.

This was confirmed when I met Linda. 'Does she not realise the stress she's putting me under and me pregnant and everything?' she said. Cara, meanwhile, sat with her eyes downcast and an impassive expression on her face. Linda went on to talk, in front of her daughter, about how Cara was always so selfish, and that, far from welcoming the new baby, she had been upset and 'stormed off' when her mum had told her about it. According to Linda, Cara had always been a quiet child whom 'you could leave to her own devices' but she had become angry and aggressive when her first half-sister was born.

I saw Cara, without her mum, for a number of sessions and she talked about how she felt her mum no longer loved her. She had always felt her mum had little time for her because she worked long hours and frequently seemed dismissive or uninterested in her. But her first real heartbreak had come when her mum had got married. She believed that Linda had chosen her step-dad over her and she had worried that she would have even less time for her then.

In fact, this was exactly what happened when her sister was born and Cara had felt even further relegated. She wasn't happy to be a big sister, but her mum had been very angry and critical of her when she showed it, calling her selfish, childish and silly. She had come to believe that she could do nothing right in her mum's eyes because now, no matter what she did, she felt blamed and criticised by her.

This seemed to me like the core of her problem. Because her mum was so critical and dismissive, Cara had come to believe she was unacceptable to her. She felt unloved and, by extension, unlovable. Her self-esteem was at rock bottom. Her suicide attempt had been a genuine attempt to kill herself because she truly believed her mother would be happier without her, especially now that a new baby was on the way.

When Cara and I eventually got her to an emotional space where she could say this to her mum, without fearing that she would be emotionally annihilated, her mum was devastated. She had had no clue about how low Cara's self-esteem had been, or how much of a role she had played in influencing that. The session was both heartbreaking and heart-warming to witness; both mother and daughter were in tears, but were talking to each other about the stuff that mattered. Hearing the truth of *her daughter's hurt and sense of rejection was transformative for Linda, who soothed some of the pain by saying sorry.*

Cara felt, for the first time, that her mum finally 'got' her and understood most of how she was feeling. Because her mum had accepted how she had felt, she could feel reassured when Linda told her how much she was loved in the family. In the months that followed, Linda worked hard to show Cara how much she was valued to help rebuild her self-esteem.

Even though it may have seemed that Cara was destined to be unhappy, to feel rejected and unacceptable, this proved not to be the case. Linda's changed attitude, becoming more positive, encouraging Cara to contribute to the family, then acknowledging and welcoming her help, showed Cara that her mum wanted and valued her. Linda used many of the tips I have included here to build Cara's self-esteem, demonstrating powerfully that children can always be helped to feel better about themselves.

Promoting self-esteem

We can build children's self-esteem and a sense that they are lovable by:

❋ **Accepting children for who they are.** We can unintentionally signal to children that they are only acceptable 'on condition ...' For example, we may suggest we want them to be smarter, thinner, more generous, quieter, better-behaved, and so on. Children need to know that we love them no matter what.

❋ **Communicating with respect.** When children make mistakes, or act in certain ways, they may be the recipients of criticism, dismissal and sarcasm. We need to let them know in how we speak to them that we believe they have valuable contributions to make.

* **Giving children undivided attention.** Attending to children individually allows them to feel special and noticed simply for being themselves.
* **Being empathetic and understanding.** When we empathise with children we help them to realise that their feelings are important and that we care about them deeply enough to notice their feelings.

We can build self-esteem and a sense of capability in children by:

* **Treating mistakes as learning opportunities.** Children, like us, are imperfect and make mistakes. Our job is to help them learn from their mistakes and avoid making similar ones, rather than being critical of their natural imperfection and using errors as a reason to punish them.
* **Giving children opportunities to contribute.** We need to let children help us and to take responsibility for different tasks. If we reject their help they will believe they are useless or ineffective. We need to let them feel they are valuable members of our family who have an important role in it, even if just as our helper.
* **Acknowledging their effort as much as their success.** In a consumerist society, the main focus is on achievement, what we have produced: the outcome over the journey. Naturally, if we never produce anything then we may feel like failures. We need to allow children to feel good about what they are doing, and their application to the task, rather than focusing only on what they achieve at the end.

- ❊ **Allowing children to make decisions and solve problems.** It is hard to feel effective and able when we have no power, or skill, to make decisions. Involving children in problem-solving and decision-making gives them a greater say in their own destiny and helps them to realise that they can do things for themselves.
- ❊ **Identifying children's strengths and abilities.** Sometimes we can assume that children know what they are good at. But if your self-esteem is low, you will discount the good stuff and probably focus more on the things you feel you fail at. To challenge any negative self-belief, we need to remind children of all the positive things about their personalities and their abilities.

The half-full glass

When we start to try to build children's self-esteem, they may seem to reject our efforts. If they have a poor self-image and a negative, hopeless outlook on life we may have to overcome a lot of inertia before they start to believe the positive things we say about them. Sometimes a negative outlook may stem from our own predominantly negative view of the world; we may have created a culture of criticism or dismissiveness based on our own experiences growing up. At others, children may have taken on board criticisms or negative beliefs about themselves from teachers, sports coaches and their peers. Bullying, for example, with repeated taunts about how children look, speak or act, may have made them feel really bad about themselves.

Indeed, if our praise and compliments are to be believable, we must show our children that we understand just how badly they see themselves, even if we don't agree with them. We may have to say something like, 'I know you think you're a bad runner but you looked like you were running your fastest in that race, which really impressed me.'

Children often tell me they don't believe their parents because 'They have to say nice stuff about me ...' so when the same positive message comes from someone else it may have more power for our children. The other thing we must remember is that our praise and positive acknowledgement must be authentic. Children will disbelieve our praise if it seems over the top, random or misplaced. If your child carries their dishes to the counter after dinner an authentic response would be, 'Thanks for bringing your dirty dishes over. It's helpful and makes one less job for me to do.' A less authentic response might be, 'Oh, you're the best, most helpful boy in the world. You're always trying to make my life easier. Thank you.' Similarly, on seeing a picture your child has painted, it may seem too much if you respond, 'You're such a wonderful artist. That's the best picture you've ever done. I'll have to put it on the fridge so everyone can see it.' A more authentic reaction may be, 'Oh, look at your picture! You worked so hard on it. I like all the reds you used. That looks like a picture to be proud of. Will we stick it on the fridge so others can see it too?'

An authentic statement that genuinely picks up on the good things will have an impact, and children come to believe good things about themselves if they hear them often enough and if they match the evidence in their behaviour or performance.

Encouraging positive self-judgement

When children achieve some success, or make a good effort, most parents will praise them or tell them they're proud of them. It's all the more powerful to say, 'Wow, you must feel so proud of yourself for ...' or 'I'd say you feel really pleased with yourself for ...'. It will encourage them to evaluate their own performance positively rather than simply receive praise from their parent, which they may discount or ignore.

Improving relationships between children to reduce sibling rivalry

As soon as our family expands beyond one child, it is likely that we will witness sibling rivalry. Think back to your own family and the relationships you had with brothers or sisters. I'm guessing there were periods when you felt hurt, anger, jealousy, distrust and suspicion about their motives or actions. There may also have been periods of support, closeness and kinship.

Despite the phrase 'blood is thicker than water', I wonder why we expect brothers and sisters to get on better than non-siblings. Simply being a brother or sister doesn't guarantee closeness or mutual respect. Positive feelings between siblings have to be nurtured, as in any other relationship.

The challenge of being a sibling

Older children lose out on their parents' time and attention when babies arrive ('Just give me a minute till I change his nappy, then I'll help you …'). Higher expectations are placed on them and their behaviour ('Don't spit your food out like the baby – you know better than that …'). They're expected to tolerate their baby sibling ('He doesn't know you were building a tower – he just wanted to help. Let him play too …'). They can lose out on personal space ('It's better for you to share the room …'). They can be expected to take on unwanted responsibility ('Keep an eye on your brother in the garden and don't let him out onto the road …').

Younger siblings may also feel that they lose out. They may not have the same freedom as older siblings or never get to do things first. They can feel in the shadow of a high-performing older child, or that their older brother or sister is more loved because they are treated specially by parents or extended family.

No matter your place in a family, you may resent what others seem to have – and end up in conflict.

Easing the arrival of a new sibling

When a baby is due, an older brother or sister may have no idea of the impact that he or she will have on them. Consequently they may be delighted and excited by the prospect of the birth, shocking us and themselves by their subsequent decline into enmity as their sibling arrives and grows into the family space.

To get things off to a positive start, when the new baby arrives you can arrange for him or her to have a gift for their brother or sister. The older sibling can be in charge of opening gifts that may come for the baby, or showing off the baby to visitors. Identify some people, like your older child's godparents, aunts, uncles or grandparents, who can make a fuss of him or her so that all of the visitors' attention isn't on the new baby.

In the early days and weeks you can try to include the older child in what is happening with the baby, as a helper or just a companion. Each parent should spend time with each child so that the older one doesn't feel they have 'lost' a parent to the baby.

Avoiding comparisons between children

It's natural to compare children; we use them as a marker for either normality or acceptability. If an older child walks at the age of one, the next child may be considered ahead or behind, depending on when they walk. If your eldest child is a whirling dervish of energy, a subsequent child may seem placid in comparison. If one child is gregarious, we may worry if the next is more introverted.

Any comment we make may unwittingly build enmity between the children. 'Your sister got her room cleaned, why haven't you?' has the potential to lead to dislike of a 'perfect' sister, while 'Why is your room not tidy yet? You've had plenty of time,' achieves the same thing with no negative comparison.

We rarely intend to compare children, but when we do so, it invariably leads one to feel that they fail (and are therefore less lovable or capable); and the other takes the blame for the sense of failure. It's easy to resent or feel jealous of someone if they always seem to do better or achieve more than you do.

The question of equality for children

Sometimes we may try to appease squabbling siblings with phrases like, 'I treat you all equally: why do you insist that things are not fair?' or 'I love you all the same, I have no favourites among you.' Although the intention behind these statements may be to reassure your children that they are equals, the reality (and their perception) is that they are not. We will seem insincere if we insist they are true.

Most of us will be angry if we feel we are the recipients of injustice. If a parent appears unfair, though, we are more likely to take out our anger on the brother or sister that has profited (unfairly, as we believe) because it may not feel safe to be angry with the parent, who may end up liking us even less. Justice and equity are big deals for lots of children. Nobody likes to feel they're getting a raw deal in the love, time, attention or treats departments.

In fact, we all love our children differently. We love different things about them. We show our love for them in different ways (some like cuddles, others don't). We can spend different amounts of time with each child or be more or less focused on one and their activities. Rather than pretending that all children are equal, it may be better to acknowledge what it is about each child that is special or that we value. This is often best done in a one-to-one. We can identify their positive traits (helpfulness, consideration, friendliness or whatever). Pointing out their specialness doesn't detract from the specialness of any other sibling.

The only thing to be alert to, while you are doing this, is that particular personality traits or repeated behaviour often mean children are assigned a particular role in the family. This is less of a problem if the trait is positive, but if the identified trait is perceived to be negative it may lead to a major issue. For example, 'Peter is the quiet one'; 'Sally is our clown, aren't you, Sally?'; 'If anyone's going to argue, it'll be Sean'. Children will take on the ascribed role, which leads them to believe they are argumentative, shy or silly.

They may feel locked into these roles and jealous of brothers and sisters who have easier, more positive or valued traits. They may also believe that if a sibling is already in a role, they can't be like that too. If, for instance, a boy hears regularly that his sister is 'the artistic one', he may believe that he is not artistic and neglect or reject his own creativity.

So, if we are going to identify what we value in our children it is important to be positive and to reassure them that this is not necessarily an exhaustive or exclusive list.

A case in point ...

Valerie and Michael were aged seven and nine respectively. Their parents, Johan and Simona, came to me despairing of their children ever getting along. The level of tension was so great that they felt their own relationship was suffering – they were rowing more. Their biggest complaint was that Michael was rough with Valerie and often hurt her. Valerie was bossy, and they also felt that sometimes she feigned hurt to get her brother into trouble. Typically they heard shouts and screams from the TV room and Valerie usually came in to them crying that Michael had hit her.

They had tried lots of things to help the children get on, such as a family outing once a week. They admitted this was often a disaster as the two didn't mind bickering and fighting in public, embarrassing their parents.

Simona couldn't understand why the children seemed to hate each other so much. She had had a great relationship with her two sisters, both of whom were older than her. Johan really sympathised with Michael, as he, too, had had 'an annoying little sister', whom he felt persecuted him, then got him into trouble whenever he reacted.

It turned out that this influenced his reaction to the children's fights to the point at which he never listened to Valerie and sided with Michael. Simona was conscious of this and felt it was unfair so she was often more sympathetic to Valerie, if she was around when a fight erupted. As they talked about this, both parents realised they were each siding with a child and acting out the conflict between the children in their own relationship.

I started the intervention by getting the parents to stop taking sides in the rows. Instead I asked them to encourage the children to sort out their differences. The technique for doing this involves the parents sitting down with the children and

- ❀ *Identifying the problem*
- ❀ *Allowing each child to say how they feel about it, then reiterating those feelings for them (for example, 'Valerie, you sound upset that Michael won't let you have a turn to choose the TV programme, and Michael, you sound angry that Valerie keeps standing in front of the TV while you're trying to watch it')*
- ❀ *Checking again that you and they have understood correctly how each feels ('So it sounds like it's upsetting to have no turn with the TV and equally upsetting to have your turn disrupted')*
- ❀ *Getting them to identify possible solutions*
- ❀ *Leaving them to choose a solution.*

In this kind of approach, parents stay involved enough to ensure that each child has seen the problem from the other perspective. They also act as the oil to keep a discussion flowing, allowing the children to be clear about what each other is saying. Critically, though, neither Johan nor Simona was allowed to make the final decision for the children about how to solve the problem.

There are times, if tempers are raised, when it can help to separate the children till they have calmed, then come back and attempt the process again.

Over time this approach yielded a successful outcome. The children realised that their parents weren't going to take over and make the decisions for them (either in their favour or not) and began to take much more notice of the impact on the other of what they did. Because their parents stayed involved, it was a constructive process, rather than destructive, as the nature of their relationship had been prior to this.

Techniques for reducing sibling rivalry

The problem-solving technique described above can be very effective in helping children to resolve some of their conflicts. Clearly, when they have fewer fights they feel less negative towards each other. Other useful ideas are:

❁ **Create time alone** for each of your children with you. This can help them realise that you value and respect them.

❁ **Don't talk about their siblings** during their time. Often we may make comments like, 'Oh, your sister would love those shoes too,' which may leave your child thinking, 'Even when she isn't here he's thinking about *her*.'

❁ **Avoid taking sides** in their disputes but show you can see both points of view.

❁ **Don't force togetherness**, especially if there is a lot of tension. Acknowledge that time apart will give them head space.

❁ **Create a mood chart.** Children don't always recognise their siblings' moods accurately and may unknowingly be antagonising an already grumpy brother or sister. It can really help younger children especially to be able to glance at a mood chart on the fridge and know what frame of mind their brother or sister is in. Using colours to represent moods, you can put their names on the fridge and they can place a square of the colour that matches their mood under their name. So, for example, green = happy, red = angry, black = worried, blue = sad. Typically, when your children come home from school, you can remind them to stick up their mood colour so that everyone else can know how they feel. If you spot, for example, that your twelve-year-old son has put a red sticker under his name, it may prompt you to find out what has angered him and warn his little brother to stay clear until your older son is feeling better.

* **Let children know what their siblings admire about them.** Often children don't realise how much or why their siblings look up to and appreciate them. This is a nice balance, too, for the vitriol they may often hear directed at them.

* **Schedule regular family meetings.** (See 'Involving children in the life and decisions of your family', page 168). These act as a forum for grievances, among other things, which can be discussed before they lead to conflict.

Children can get on with each other, but sometimes things don't work. Empathising with their feelings of hurt, upset and even hate can reduce the amount of enmity they show and may help their relationship to blossom instead.

Thriving within the school gates

Going to school is a testing time for children. They come under new social and academic pressures, and for some families it is the first time we get any inkling that our children may have a problem. We want them to thrive within their new school environment but we have to accept that we can do little to control or regulate their experience there. We have to 'let them go' as they walk through the school gates.

Two major issues likely to concern families during the primary-school years are homework and bullying. Giving our children the skills and confidence to deal with these things may take many hours of family time over the course of their school lives. Reflecting their importance, I have dealt with them fully in their own sections in Chapters 5 and 6 respectively.

The impact of home life on school life

We usually think of school and home as two distinct environments, and to some degree, they are. Different rules and expectations apply and children have to learn how to behave in each place. What we sometimes forget, however, is that our children are the common factor that links the two settings; they will carry back and forth what happens in each. For example, if your son received extra homework for messing in class, you can be sure he'll arrive home in a bad mood. That mood might be even worse if he felt unfairly punished. The atmosphere for your evening at home may be so influenced by it that your whole family will feel the knock-on effect of his misbehaviour at school.

Similarly, stuff that goes on at home will affect how they do in school. Significant events, like parental conflict or separation, custody and access disputes, bereavements, financial stress, moving house, having a sibling with a disability, a new baby arriving, parents' work pressures and family illness will all have an effect on your child.

Almost any situation that places parents or families under stress has the potential to unsettle a child. If they are worried or anxious, they may be unable to concentrate and fall behind academically. If they are stressed, they may be quick to anger, which may lead to conflict with other pupils. Their behaviour may frustrate their teacher, who loses patience with them, and a cycle of negative interaction may begin, with your child labelled a 'messer'. Any label or reputation a child earns early in their school career has the potential to follow them through that school.

A case in point ...

Sean was an eleven-year-old in fifth class at primary school. He lived with his mum and younger sister. His parents had been separated for about a year by the time he came to meet me. Prior to that, their relationship had been troubled, with lots of rows, including some physical fights. Sean was having major difficulties in school where he and his male teacher were at loggerheads; he had been threatened with exclusion from school for disruptive and threatening behaviour, which was when his mum brought him to me.

I was struck by how angry and resistant he was. He didn't want to be meeting a psychologist. He was fed up with school, fed up with his mum, and thought the whole thing was a waste of time. It took two sessions before Sean really opened up about his feelings, and when he did his real pain and distress were evident.

Although he had a tough, 'I don't care' exterior, the truth was that he did care. He cared deeply about his dad and missed him terribly. His dad hadn't been great at staying in touch since he had left home, and Sean blamed his mum for forcing his dad to go. He was really angry about them separating. He acknowledged that their house had been a stressful place to live with all of the fighting, but his parents' separation hadn't reduced the fighting. It just meant his dad was less available. Whenever his parents did meet or talk on the phone it still ended in a blazing row.

Sean was constantly rowing with his mother, for whom he had little respect. She was also negative about Sean and considered him 'pig-headed and argumentative, just like his father'. She believed that he had inherited his father's angry streak. In fact, she eventually admitted that when she was fighting with Sean she was often thinking about his dad.

Sean hated his current teacher who, according to him, 'tries to be a hard-ass'. He believed that his teacher had it in for him and that, no matter what he did in school, he was going to get into trouble. He didn't think anyone in the school cared about him, *then corrected himself: the resource teacher (whom he went to any time he was 'kicked out' of class) was lovely to him. It turned out he spent some time of every day with this person.*

I felt that Sean's difficulties in school were predated by the amount of conflict he had witnessed at home. He had been burying his feelings of stress, fear and anger for years. This year he was faced with a very authoritarian teacher and he had reacted, letting out the pent-up anger and becoming aggressive in school.

Understanding why Sean was so angry helped the school to take a new perspective on him. Once his teacher realised that Sean wasn't simply challenging him, he took a much more empathetic approach in dealing with him. The principal arranged for Sean to have some planned time out of class each day for 'project work' with the resource teacher.

Over time Sean became less angry and provocative. Gradually his parents changed how they approached each other, and once their conflict diminished, Sean no longer felt he had to take sides or feel trapped in the middle of their rows. His mum was finally able to acknowledge that her decision to tell his dad to leave had had an unintended but strong negative impact on her son. She also saw that he wasn't a carbon copy of his dad and that she shouldn't act out with Sean her issues with her husband. Meanwhile, Sean's dad accepted that he needed to be a regular and reliable influence on Sean, spending lots of time with him.

How we as parents relate to the school

If all is well with our children in school, we will probably have little interaction with their teachers or the principal. However, once any issues arise we may find ourselves frequent visitors to the school. It is amazing how powerfully being in a principal's office can jog our memories. Our own experiences of school, whether we liked, abhorred or tolerated it, will influence our interactions with teachers and principals when we meet them as parents.

Many of us will have memories of corporal punishment in school and of being beaten or humiliated there. Perhaps they are balanced by good ones too, of inspirational teachers, or a principal who showed caring and understanding. Whatever our experience, though, it will be rekindled by a formal meeting in a school. We need to be alert to this, especially if our experience was bad. We may have to override our memories in order to be open-minded and hear what our child's teachers have to tell us about him or her. If our child can benefit from extra help that a school can provide, it's important that we open ourselves to this and avoid letting latent hostility get in the way.

Schools are systems, with many layers of complex relationships that must be considered in dealing with situations. Decisions that are made, or incidents that occur, can affect a wide range of people. This means that the principal you meet about your child will have an eye to everyone in the class or the school. We have the comparative luxury of being interested only in our child. It helps, therefore, if we can keep in mind the needs of the other 'stakeholders' in the school.

Even in situations with teachers and principals who reject challenges to their views, it is still important to see beyond our own perspective. Pushing too hard about a single issue may affect the working relationship we need to maintain with our child's teacher and the school. If we approach conflict resolution in an aggressive, unreasonable or threatening way, we can expect to encounter greater resistance from the school, which may become defensive or even retaliatory. This won't help our child, who may even end up more targeted as a result of our behaviour.

Our goal is to be assertive in ensuring that our child's needs are met, while understanding the challenges and difficulties that this may present to other members of the school community.

'Stakeholders': people who have an involvement in school

* Pupils: each has a right and a responsibility to learn
* Teachers: each has a right and a responsibility to teach
* Principals: charged with managing every aspect of the day-to-day running of the school
* Parents: required to support the activities of the school
* Boards of management: charged with strategic management of the school and upholding the ethos of the school
* Patron body: responsible for determining the ethos of the school
* Department of Education and Skills: responsible for core funding of the school and determining overall policies and standards that schools must attain.

Understanding common learning difficulties

Learning difficulties can affect how children listen, think, store, retrieve, write, read and communicate information.

* **Visual perception disability:** this may cause your child to reverse or rotate letters and numbers or to be unable to focus on specific letters and words on a page. When children start formal learning of letters and numbers, reversals and rotations are common, up to around the age of seven.
* **Auditory perception disability:** similar words may sound alike and cause confusion, or a child may be unable to process words as fast as people are speaking them.

* **Sensory integration difficulties:** the child's brain may struggle to make sense of the sensory information (vision, touch, balance) it receives.
* **Gross and fine motor skills issues:** gross motor skills include walking or using a racquet to hit a ball. Fine motor skills include dexterity with the fingers in holding a pencil.
* **Sequencing disabilities:** a child may confuse the sequence of words and letters, or numbers in maths problems.
* **Organisational difficulties:** a child may find it hard to plan ahead, running out of space on a page, or failing to have the right books ready for a subject lesson.
* **Specific learning disabilities:** also called dyslexia, which appears as specific delay in reading, writing or arithmetic, despite average or above average overall ability.
* **Expressive difficulties:** some children have difficulty in expressing themselves, through speech, writing or drawing.

Most children with learning difficulties, or disabilities, have one or more of the above problems, affecting how they input, integrate or output information. Some children always have difficulty in learning new things, while others do well in school at first, but start to have problems as the challenges they face become more advanced.

Unrecognised learning difficulties have a huge impact on how a child is perceived. Often he or she is blamed for poor performance over which they have little control. Once teachers and even other pupils realise that there is an explanation for why a child is struggling academically or socially they become more tolerant, and perhaps more accepting of a different standard of work or interaction.

Identifying or diagnosing difficulties will, ultimately, be the parents' responsibility but in practice this is often done in conjunction with the child's school. Hopefully communication between you and your child's school will mean that you hear promptly about any difficulties a teacher may observe, or that you can bring your own observations to the teacher. On the basis of your discussions with the school, you may agree to have a formal psychological assessment of your child carried out to determine the nature and extent of any problems.

The Department of Education and Skills co-ordinates the National Educational Psychology Service (NEPS) and schools are entitled to a limited number of psychological assessments, by NEPS, in each academic year. Where possible, they will try to arrange the assessment of your child, but sometimes their allocation will have been used so parents must go for the private alternative.

Parents can arrange an assessment by contacting an educational or clinical psychologist. NEPS has a list of those in private practice who are eligible to carry out assessments on their behalf, so you should ensure that any psychologist you choose has NEPS approval and is on the list. You can see the approved Panel of Psychologists online by visiting the Department of Education and Skills website and following the links for NEPS.

An assessing psychologist may recommend specific assessment of your child by an occupational or speech and language therapist for sensory, motor or language issues. They should also make a range of recommendations for additional school-based support (if needed) and other teaching strategies that you and the school can implement to help.

Common behavioural difficulties

Sometimes behavioural difficulties emerge as a child tries to mask their inability to perform academic tasks, or because they feel a failure in comparison with others in the class. Children can easily lose their motivation to work or pay attention in class when they feel there is no point. They may distract other children, or be giddy or disruptive to escape the challenges that learning poses.

Sometimes other issues are identified as causing your child's problems:

❁ **Attention Deficit Disorder (ADD):** characterised by a child who is impulsive, inattentive, lacking in concentration, distractible, careless, heedless and disorganised.

* **Attention Deficit Hyperactivity Disorder (ADHD):**
  as ADD, but with giddiness, inability to sit still and
  hyperactive behaviour.
* **Oppositional Defiant Disorder (ODD):** the child is
  consistently defiant, stubborn, provocative, argumentative,
  blaming, resentful, and loses their temper easily.
* **Conduct Disorder (CD):** characterised by a child with
  severe anti-social behaviour like stealing, bullying,
  aggression, violently and intentionally hurting others,
  including animals, and fire-setting.

I don't like to pigeonhole children according to these categories
as I fear that others won't see past the label to meet the needs of the
child.

Almost invariably, however, if your child is struggling with their
behaviour in school they will be struggling just as much at home
and in other environments like sports clubs. If it is only at school
that they behave badly, perhaps something about the responses of
the adults there (or the other pupils) is causing them to react in this
way. A child who fights in school may be being bullied, for example.
A child who is in conflict with their teacher may be struggling with
a personality clash or to cope with their particular discipline style.

As with learning difficulties, your child's school is likely to
contact you about behavioural issues and may seek a psychological
assessment of your child that should try to quantify the nature of the
difficulties and propose possible interventions to help. It is during
this kind of assessment that issues like ADHD may be identified.

If an assessment suggests that your child may have ADHD or
ODD then he or she is likely to be referred for specialised assessment
to your local HSE Child and Adolescent Mental Health Service
(CAMHS). Assuming that the waiting list is not insurmountable,
engagement with CAMHS will hopefully be able to explain how
and why the difficult behaviour has developed and what you and/or
your child can do to address it.

Helping the family: the value of chores in learning about responsibility

I love chores for children. I like to share the workload involved in keeping a home and family going. If there's less for me to do, I'm more likely to feel I can stop and relax sometimes. When my children do chores, I don't resent having to do housework because everyone in the family is doing their bit.

It's not unusual to hate housework. I get no pleasure from it and do it because it needs to be done. There is a greater sense of equity amid the daily (often thankless) tasks when everyone does a share according to their ability. Most importantly, dividing house- or garden work between us means we share the responsibility for keeping our family ticking over.

Children need to learn to share the responsibility for household tasks when they are young as a precursor to taking responsibility for their own family in the future. Parents will naturally take the greatest (and final) responsibility for jobs. It's part of what we sign up for when we create a family who depend on us. However, that dependence is not eternal and if children are to grow to independence they need to know how to look after themselves and others.

I'm not a slave-driver, but I do want my children to know that we all have to pull together for our family to thrive. Children need to be involved in a wide range of family activities, which include keeping the house clean, tidy(ish) and welcoming.

A case in point ...

Emma had four children and was exhausted. She felt she spent her whole day at her children's beck and call, cooking, cleaning and washing clothes. Meanwhile she felt tormented by the constant noise in the house: arguing, loud music, excited games, racing around, tumbles, injuries, claims of starvation; even the children's laughter grated on her. Emma felt she never had a break from them. She hated the chaos and drudgery of her house, and while she acknowledged that she loved her children, she regularly felt she didn't like them.

It wasn't the first time I had come across such profound disillusionment in a parent. It turned out that Emma had expected a lot more support from her husband when they had first had children. In reality he worked such long hours in a financially rewarding job that he wasn't present enough to help practically with rearing the children and running the household. Emma had never felt able to challenge this because she valued his salary and accepted the hours he put in to earn it.

Emma had grown up as the third child, but only girl, of four children. Her mother had stayed at home to bring them up and her father had come home every evening at 5.45. 'You could set a clock by him,' she said. She also recalled that her father rarely seemed to do anything when he got in, other than eat the dinner that was served to him, read the paper and watch the nine o'clock news. She didn't remember him being particularly involved in any of their lives, even though he was always there.

She resented her three brothers because she felt they did nothing (and were asked to do nothing) around the house. Like her father, the boys seemed to have some protected status where chores were concerned. Meanwhile Emma was expected to help her mother. While she hated the unequal division of labour in the house she also, it seemed, accepted this script for how families should function.

Now, in her own family with her husband, she resented being alone with the housework and rearing the children but didn't challenge the status quo and seemed grudgingly to accept it. Understanding this dynamic was helpful for Emma; she realised that she had essentially accepted being taken for granted. It was her resentment of her role that had led to her frustration with and dislike of the children. It was as if their chaotically selfish lives were a constant reminder of the injustice she felt about her lot in life.

I encouraged Emma to discuss all of this with her husband, whom she acknowledged probably had no clue about her stress and distress. Clearly, being alone in the parenting of four children was taking its toll on her and she needed him to share some of that burden.

To try to regain some order, and better balance, in the family Emma set up two weekly planners. One contained all of the activities the children did after school. In writing it, she was forced to reconsider the breadth of things they did; then she sat down with the whole family to rationalise what was achievable, and each child chose one activity to forgo. The second planner listed the household tasks and assigned chores to the children (and her husband) that they all needed to achieve by each Friday night. The jobs weren't onerous: they involved setting the table, tidying up after dinner, emptying and filling the dishwasher, keeping clothes off bedroom floors, tidying each bedroom weekly, and so on. Receipt of pocket money depended on tasks having been done. Emma committed herself to helping any of the children with their chores until they knew what to do and how to do it.

It was too idealistic to hope that the whole house would be transformed overnight. Nonetheless, Emma shifted the dynamic enough that her husband acknowledged the stress she was under and became more involved in rearing the children, coming home early two nights a week to help ferry them to activities.

She also noticed how effective sharing the chores was in re-energising everyone and gaining their respect. She admitted it was hard to motivate the children at first because they were so unused to helping but, with her constant involvement, momentum grew and some chores became pure habit for the children. She didn't mind the energy it took to kick-start them because she finally felt appreciated and valued when everyone realised how much she had been doing. Of course, the children grumbled about having to work but she noticed that they then showed real pride in what they had achieved.

The children still fought regularly, but Emma didn't mind so much because she no longer felt exhausted and had the energy to try to help the children understand each other's perspectives and opinions.

Children don't need to 'want' to do chores

Helping out around the house is not usually the kind of thing a child volunteers for so they take on the responsibility because they have no choice. Eventually, performing the task becomes a habit. In later years, they may come to see the intrinsic value of the work, by which stage they will probably also have a well-developed sense of responsibility. In their earlier years, however, it is enough that they do the work; they don't need to like it! Grumbling and complaining children who sweep the floor or clear the dinner table are better than children who skive off to the TV or the computer.

Establishing the habit of chores

When children are in their toddler years, they naturally show a desire to help us in whatever tasks we're doing. If we cook, for example, they may push a chair to the counter, wanting to stir, chop or mash (or taste!), shell peas or 'help' in some way. It is only as time passes that their interest fades. Sometimes this is down to us: we give off signals that we are too busy to devote the time to their 'helping'. It requires a lot of vigilance and patience to do jobs with a toddler or pre-schooler in tow. Sometimes we let them know that they create more mess than assistance so they aren't welcome. At others they find alternative ways to occupy their time and we are left 'helperless'.

By the time children go to school the helping habit may already have been lost. Also, we tend to be more protective then of their energy; after homework is done we may want to avoid overloading them with jobs. However, most children have plenty of energy left after school and homework and certainly enough for short household tasks.

Habit and routine are the strongest predictors of children's future chore participation. If we can begin early, with the assumption that children will be involved according to their capacity, we can instil the notion that doing chores is part of the natural order at home. So, take advantage of your toddler's desire to help you and keep the helping going.

Ideas to get children activated in the house

* Chores should not be overwhelming. Be realistic and bear your child's age in mind. Examples might include carrying dishes from table to sink for young children and making their bed for the older ones.
* Don't forget to teach, or demonstrate regularly, how a job should be done.
* Involve your child in determining the tasks he or she will complete, perhaps by holding a quick meeting each week to discuss what needs to be done and who will do it.
* Create a weekly chore chart to remind everyone of what they're doing and to note when the jobs get done.
* Rotate the tasks every week so that children don't get bored or feel stuck with 'hard' or unpleasant jobs.
* Give lots of encouragement, praise and support for the work that gets done, bearing in mind the principle that putting in the effort is more important than the final result.
* By working alongside your children you instil in them the concept that everyone is pulling together for the good of the family.

The phrase 'helping the family' is a nice one to use when introducing the idea of chores. It gives a child a clear indication that they are not doing us a favour in clearing the table or emptying the dishwasher, rather that they are performing a really useful and valued role.

Feeling able and useful supports self-esteem. Children who have the satisfaction of taking on responsibility for work in the family, which they know is valued and appreciated, will have higher self-esteem. All of the research shows that children with high self-esteem thrive.

Benefits of children doing chores

Research also shows that children involved in household chores are likely to do well in adult life (it's more important in determining their success even than their parents' interaction style or their own intelligence). They are more likely to complete their education, determine a career for themselves, enjoy close and warm relationships with others, and less likely to resort to drug use. It's remarkable but true, and proves the clear benefit to children of doing chores even when many other variables, such as parenting styles, gender, types of household task, time spent on tasks, attitudes and motivators associated with doing the tasks and intelligence, are taken into consideration.

Even though we parents have to put in some effort to get our children to participate in household tasks, the benefits well outweigh it.

Involving children in the life and decisions of your family

Family meetings are a great way to involve children in the decision-making aspects of family life. They give every member an opportunity to listen respectfully to everyone else's view on a range of issues that affect us all, especially as your children get older, and their schedule often becomes as busy as your own. In practice we may only get to chat with our children at family meals or in brief moments, perhaps while going to bed or on the way to and from an activity.

Those times aren't really conducive to dealing with the nitty-gritty of issues that emerge, and we may skate over the surface of stuff that has been going on without really understanding it. This is where scheduled family meetings come in.

There is no specific formula or agenda for family meetings. They can cover any number of topics. Typically families choose to look at whatever is happening in a given week, the things that have been going well or badly within the family, or any grievances individuals may have. Sometimes a meeting may be about something that needs to be changed or improved, even about congratulating ourselves on our achievements or successes as a family.

Because family meetings are a deliberately protected space in the week they have a different status for children from regular chats or even dinner-table discussions. They make children feel like integral members of the family, which they appreciate, because they have an opportunity to air grievances, help to make family plans and be involved in decisions.

Family meetings will look different in every family, given the range of ages that are present. At the early stages of family life the quality of the discussions may not feel very productive or even very inclusive, but by starting early we can institute a habit that will reap rewards when the children are older and the need to discuss issues respectfully will be greater. If we introduce family meetings when the children are older, we may find that the initial meetings are about setting ground rules and ensuring that the discussions are fruitful, rather than turning into opportunities for conflict, contempt and hurt.

How to structure family meetings

First, establish (and keep) a time each week at which all the family are available. We need to tell our children the rationale for the meetings, which is that they will improve communication, connect the family, and allow everyone to share what is going on in their lives.

There is no set age at which to begin family meetings. They can work well, if the subject matter is pitched at an appropriate level, with children as young as five or six. Generally, though, families find that they become more useful as life gets busier and children are seven or eight.

At the start the meetings will be driven and co-ordinated by us, the parents, but depending on the age of your children, they can be led later by each family member in turn. It is a good idea, too, to appoint a minute-taker to note down any decisions that are made and agreed. I find that ground rules about listening, not interrupting, being honest and contributing help the flow and underline the core respect for each person and their contribution(s).

If you take it in turns to speak, it becomes clear that everyone will have a chance to put their point of view about each topic and that everyone's contribution is valued. So, for example, everyone can share a good thing that happened to them in the week and a difficulty they faced. If you are problem-solving, everyone gets a turn to suggest a solution (like a brainstorming session) before any judgements are made or the suggestions refined. Parents can always smooth things over, if need be, even if they're not the leader for the day, by praising the good listening they observe, empathising with difficulties or thanking people for their contributions.

A typical agenda

When children are younger, parents are likely to drive family meetings so are more likely to set the agenda. We can encourage each child to raise any issue they may have and can then determine the decision. When children reach the age of ten, perhaps, and have experienced several family meetings, they can successfully run one by following an agenda, with our support to make sure everyone's voice is heard.

Here is a typical agenda from a family who had monthly meetings. They comprised Mum and Dad, Miriam, aged thirteen, Robert, eleven, and Sammy, seven.

April 2012 Meeting

Meeting boss: Miriam

Helper: Dad

Agenda:

1. Good things that have happened since March meeting

2. Problems that have happened since March meeting

3. Things that we must agree on:

   - Robert wants his own bedroom

   - Sammy wants chocolate spread included in the weekly shopping

   - Will the children get to do a summer camp each this summer?

   - How to share out the TV fairly (Miriam thinks Robert hogs it)

   - Updating the chore list since Sammy can now do more things

4. Recording the decisions

In this family the 'helper' is always either Mum or Dad and they record the final decisions. The record of the April meeting was stuck on the fridge and looked like this:

Good things:

1. Dad booked his holidays from work for the first two weeks in July.

2. Mum got €600 from Granny who was left money in Great Aunt Sarah's will.
3. Miriam got picked for the county under-14 camogie panel.
4. Robert got a prize in his school poetry competition.
5. Sammy scored a goal in his first soccer game of the season.

Problems:
1. Fighting over the TV remote is out of hand.
2. The toilet in the upstairs bathroom doesn't flush properly so everyone has to use the loo under the stairs till we can get it fixed. Please read the sign that reminds you of this!!!

Decisions we made:
1. Robert can't have his own room yet because we have nowhere else to store the junk in the box room. But we will find out how much it'll cost to get folding stairs fitted to the attic hatch so that stuff can be stored there instead.
2. Chocolate spread is our holiday treat and the majority of us want to keep it that way so we are not buying it every week.
3. The money we got from the will (thanks, Granny!) means each child can pick a summer camp to do and must tell Mum before the end of April so she can book them.
4. Miriam will make a TV Watching Chart where people can book a time to watch their preferred programme each day (we can record any programmes that overlap). The TV will only be allowed on from 4 p.m. to 6 p.m. on schooldays and this can be increased if the chart helps everyone to agree whose turn it is and the fighting stops.
5. Sammy agreed to start sweeping the kitchen floor after meals so Miriam will now vacuum the whole house once a fortnight instead of sweeping the kitchen floor. Robert will continue to wipe down the table after meals and everyone still takes turns emptying the dishwasher. Mum will do a new Chore List and stick it up on the kitchen whiteboard.

A case in point ...

Norma was a stay-at-home mum to four children, aged seven, nine, ten and thirteen. She also minded two other children, aged three and seven, three days a week. She contacted me in May one year because she was dreading the school holidays. For Norma, holiday time meant impending mayhem.

Norma was conscious that the noise levels in the house were extreme at times and she found herself shouting, roaring and screaming 'like a lunatic' just to be heard among the chaos. She described it as a constant battle in her house, with all four children being very demanding in their own ways. It felt to Norma that their lives were a constant drama full of passion and incident. She reckoned that her husband was the only calm person in the house. I remembered her plea to me: 'If only we could be civil to each other ...'

In many ways their family life sounded normal in as much as six children up to the age of thirteen would make any house busy and noisy. It is possible to have a calm family environment, but not exclusively so. All children need opportunities to vent their energy and that means they will, on occasion, get very excitable, dramatic, loud and busy. If we accept that some noise and chaos is unavoidable, we can be more realistic in achieving a bit of calm.

I got Norma and Brian to imagine themselves as their ten-year-old daughter and asked them what she wanted or needed. Each identified some variation on the theme of a proper space or time to talk, without interruption or competition. That was exactly what we decided to create in their family. Because the children were all old enough, I felt that a designated family meeting, at least weekly, would allow many of the children's issues to be aired, but in a setting where everybody had a voice and Brian and Norma could help the children to develop their listening skills.

The important thing, I felt, was that each child was listened to independently. Part of the clamour in the house seemed to result from everyone vying for attention all the time. In the usual chaos it was often the child who shouted loudest who was heard. Equally, many of the children's views were lost or ignored, to the point at which they might easily feel they were not important to their parents.

Family meetings had the real benefit of according each child equal weight and value, helping to build their self-respect, as well as their ability to listen to and respect each other. Friday evenings were one of the few times when everyone was around so this became the designated family meeting time. Because the meeting needed to happen early they decided to follow it with a takeaway meal from the local Indian restaurant. They were lucky to be able to afford this luxury, which took pressure off Norma and Brian, who didn't have to worry about cooking and were able to devote the time to the children. It was also a nice reward for the children after they had participated fully in the meeting.

In a follow-up appointment three months later, Norma confirmed that the meetings had been a turning point in the family dynamic. They had set their rules as I'd suggested, and heavily invested in supporting the children to listen to each other, by commenting on and praising each child for eye contact with the speaker, lack of interruption, proper turn-taking, a sibling expanding on the view of a previous speaker, or any other sign that they were paying attention to each other.

The range of issues the children brought up was fascinating, from how they organised homework (their eldest asking for his own quiet space to study) to the many sibling rivalries, Brian's smoking (everyone was worried he would get lung cancer) and the family policy on recycling (the nine-year-old pushed for a bin so they could segregate their waste, as happened at school). Mostly, though, the meetings created a respectful space in the week that the children came to appreciate and to extend into more of their interactions with each other. For sure there were still tears, occasional tantrums, minor traumas and heated *disagreements, but the piercing intensity and chaos seemed to have gone.*

Why democracy promotes family harmony with older children

The family meeting is a deceptively powerful mechanism to promote family harmony. In the first instance, it makes explicit the need for good communication. When things are a bit frantic it's easy to forget to say important things or to miss opportunities to influence decisions. If we find that we have fallen into negative cycles of interaction, we may also have slipped into a 'top-down' style of communicating where we lay down the law, make all the decisions, then simply inform our children of them.

At times we do this because it seems expedient and we don't want argument and dissent. In the longer term, however, dictatorial decision-making tells our children that their views and opinions don't count, that we don't respect them or their ideas. The family meeting opens a forum for our children's voices to be heard and to have greater influence, building their self-respect and belief that they have something valuable to contribute.

Moaning and complaining have a role, too!

We may feel that encouraging dissent and differing opinion may be destabilising or destructive to the fabric of our family, but in fact the opposite is true. When children or parents have to hold back their frustrations or feelings of inequity, their hurt or disagreement, such feelings tend to fester emotionally.

Bad feelings are invariably expressed, but if there is no forum to express them directly about the issue that has caused them, they may be expressed indirectly, through tantrums, arguments or other conflict.

> If you encourage children to voice their negative feelings when they can be dealt with empathetically, and responded to compassionately, you will support their emotional development and reduce tension and conflict in the home.

Family meetings and problem-solving

Problem-solving is a skill that we learn. Children may or may not naturally develop strategies to solve problems, but if we hear them saying, 'I can't …' or 'There's no point …' it's quite likely that they need help to overcome a difficulty. Sometimes it's tempting, for expediency's sake, to step in and resolve the issue for them. However, if we continuously solve their problems, they will never learn to do it themselves.

Imagine your eleven-year-old son stomping into the kitchen to complain that he can't play soccer today because his shin-guards are too small and the coach won't let him play unless he wears them. He may be angry that he'll miss a match, or blaming you because he doesn't have new ones. A typical reaction may have us telling him not to be 'such a drama queen', and then, in an I-don't-know-why-you-couldn't-think-of-this-yourself tone, suggesting he text his friend (whom you know is sick) to borrow his shin-guards for the day.

While the suggestion may solve the problem, it doesn't help our boy to learn how to solve a similar problem. A different approach to his initial moan might be to empathise that this does sound tricky since he really wants to play but is missing a vital piece of kit. We can ask him what he might do about it. We can prompt him to consider different options, like going to a shop to buy a new pair, borrowing a pair, putting up with the discomfort of his current shin-guards one last time. Then we can help him to work out the pros and cons of each option and to refine the seemingly best solution (if he decides to borrow a pair, help him work out whom best to borrow from).

Working through a problem-solving process in this way allows him to learn the steps so that he can do it for himself another time.

Family meetings are a fertile resource for identifying problems and demonstrating how we can solve them:

1. Specify exactly what the problem is.
2. Brainstorm possible solutions.
3. Evaluate the likely outcomes of these solutions.
4. Decide on a solution that seems to offer the best chance of success.
5. Review the solution we chose afterwards, to learn if there may be a better approach to take the next time we have a similar problem.

Although we may never have broken down the process like this, we know intuitively that this is how we solve problems. This process becomes automatic. We know it from observing others dealing with problems and from trying to grapple with them ourselves. Are we always conscious that this is the process we undergo when faced with a problem? Probably not. That is why, in family meetings, we can become more explicit about the steps that need to be taken in solving a problem. And by involving our children, we can increase the pool of potential solutions. Also, they are more likely to enact the solutions when they feel they have contributed to arriving at them. Again, feeling part of the process supports a child's self-esteem since they can feel capable and successful if they overcome what seemed an insurmountable difficulty.

Children will also feel respected when they are involved in the decisions that affect them. Whether they are big decisions, like moving house or selecting a secondary school, or small ones, like choosing what kind of takeaway to get for the monthly treat night, children feel better when they have a say. We don't need to pander to them or always agree to their solutions or opinions; we can still make the final decision because families are not necessarily run democratically. Nevertheless, including them makes them feel better about themselves. If children feel respected, they are much more likely to respect us, and others, in return.

Making sense of the media that influences your children

Televisions, computer games and the Internet are ever present and have insinuated themselves into the heart of our family lives. Many families have more than one TV, and either cable or satellite connection to hundreds of stations. Most have at least one gaming system, like the Wii, Xbox or PlayStation, as well as several handheld gaming devices or smartphones. Most homes will be connected to the Internet with a router to spread the connection to multiple devices, like games consoles, phones, desktop computers, laptops or tablets. Many houses will also have a radio on in the background and newspapers strewn about. Through all of these media, we expose our children to multiple, and at times competing, influences beyond the messages we want to give them about our values and beliefs.

Let's not kid ourselves that we barely use the technology and media at our disposal. Research shows that, increasingly, children spend at least forty hours a week engaged with some form of digital media (including TV, computer games, mobile phones and Internet-based social networking). That equates to between six and seven hours of media consumption every day. In other words, our children are spending almost all their free time plugged into a digital world. That is time not spent on homework, reading, purely socialising, being with the family or playing outside.

There is a mounting body of evidence that the balance in children's lives between activities that stimulate their brains and their bodies is awry. Indeed, the sedentary nature of their lives, directly linked to sitting in front of a TV or monitor, is associated with overweight and the development of Type II diabetes. High levels of TV-watching and computer-gaming are also associated with disrupted sleep or difficulty in falling asleep. When children play computer games just before bed it has an especially marked effect on how long it takes them to drop off.

Research shows that between 93 and 98 per cent of children and teenagers play video games on the Internet, directly on their computer, phones or games consoles. The amount varies according to different studies but children and teenagers will play, on average, between fourteen and twenty hours of computer or video games per week – about half of their total digital consumption.

Lots of us struggle with demands for new video games because we resent the amount of time our children spend in front of the TV and games console or the computer. We also struggle with the games children ask for; many of the most popular ones are eighteen-rated yet are played by younger groups. Many parents feel isolated as they resist certain games in the face of mounting frustration from their pre-teen or early-teen child who complains, 'All my friends have it and play it!'

The same pressure applies to mobile phones. With smartphone technology getting cheaper, even entry-level phones can have Wi-Fi Internet connectivity and/or unlimited data use. Televisions have Internet connectivity built in. Our children will harangue us with tales of how much time or access their friends get to these media and the underlying message is that if we try to restrict them in any way we will hamper them socially.

Mind you, some of the access that children have to media is facilitated and indeed welcomed by parents. As we worry more about the dangers our children may face in the world, it suits many of us to know that they are safely at home. The ease with which this technology has entered our lives stems from many parents' desire for their children to be occupied without them. Let's be honest, most of us are busy and it suits us to have our children plugged into a games console or the TV because it saves us having to entertain or supervise them. At least we can get a load of washing on or the dinner cooked without too much interruption. We can opt for what seems to be the easier life.

But what is the true cost of those forty hours' digital exposure for our children? Its potential influence on their development and behaviour is as yet largely unexplored, but I believe this level of exposure could impact significantly on them. We have all come across children who seem to carry what we often describe as a sense of entitlement. They appear to think their every whim should be granted, and kick up a fuss if it isn't. Parents wishing to avoid conflict by indulging their offspring may be contributing to this behaviour but it develops in part because the global media strongly influences our children to seek what they want when they want and how they want it.

Whether it be explicit advertising campaigns targeted at children for fast food, toys or clothes, or implicit messages from music videos, TV programmes and the like, our children receive many different messages about what is available to them. This increases their sense of expectation and creates demand or desire in them. Within the broad range of media they see other children with particular brands of clothes or living particular lifestyles and they want them too. These influences are far broader and more potentially persuasive than those of our children's peer group; they can lead children to become more demanding, adding to the pressures on parents.

I believe we have a responsibility as parents to regulate and monitor our children's access to TV, the Internet, computer- and video-gaming. Every family will have a different view on how much media they want to allow into their lives. In practice, if you start off by being restrictive with your toddlers, you will find that as they get older and more connected to friends, you have to adapt, probably increasing the amount of time in front of a screen or what they can do online. It's always easier to loosen the reins, so to speak, than to tighten them, and you may find that you strike a better balance if you keep them away from digital media in their early years.

A case in point ...

Richard and Monica had three children, aged three, five and nine, all boys. They came to see me because of their eldest boy.

He was struggling in school to concentrate and was forever in trouble for distracting other children, then reacting aggressively when reprimanded. The school also felt he was too boisterous and rough in the playground. Richard and Monica had been in to meet the principal three times already that year. She had given them an ultimatum to have him assessed as the teacher needed additional support to manage him; the school could only apply for a special needs assistant on the basis of a psychological assessment. I explained to the Browns that I don't carry out that kind of assessment but they asked to meet me anyway while they were waiting for an appointment with another psychologist.

I asked the Browns many questions about their family, focusing especially on Brendan, the eldest. I was particularly interested in whether he showed the same distractibility and poor concentration at home. It turned out that he struggled with his homework but his parents had noticed that he was well able to concentrate on his computer games or if he was watching a TV programme he enjoyed. Brendan was plugged into the TV or the games console for hours every evening and at the weekends.

Richard and Monica rarely set any limits on TV or computer-game time since Brendan and the other two seemed to enjoy them. Also, they kept the boys occupied and stopped them fighting too much. It was not uncommon for Brendan to come home and start straight into watching TV while he had a snack. There was war when his mum tried to get him away from the TV to sit down to do his homework. As soon as he had finished it he was back to the TV until dinner. The set stayed on in the background all through the evening.

I didn't assume there was no other explanation for Brendan's behaviour. He may have had Attention Deficit Hyperactivity Disorder, but his TV and gaming habits seemed hugely important in his subsequent behaviour. Richard and Monica had noticed that he always seemed more hyper and aggressive after a couple of hours at his favourite wrestling game on the console. He frequently tried to wrestle his little brother, listing his 'moves' as he performed them.

The Browns had a six-week wait for Brendan's assessment and I encouraged them to try an experiment during that time. Their task was to switch off the TV and games console during the week and to limit TV or game time to four hours in total over the weekend. They were horrified at the thought of how they could introduce or enforce such a ban. They anticipated an angry and abusive backlash from Brendan and his siblings.

I agreed that in the early days he might be very upset and that he would require a heavy investment of their time until he learned how to occupy himself with toys or books instead of the TV and games console. But I was able to reassure them that if they could, responsibly, stick by their guns, he would come to accept the new family rules.

It turned out that it was, indeed, really hard for Monica and Richard to implement the media ban, but ultimately worthwhile. Within the six weeks while they waited for the assessment, Brendan's behaviour began to settle in school and his aggression diminished. Either Richard or Monica tried to make themselves available to the children in the evenings to structure or scaffold their play as need be.

When Brendan was assessed he was found to have no behavioural disorders, but he did have a specific learning difficulty (dyslexia). It had made school a struggle for Brendan and he had often felt he was failing or stupid because he couldn't learn as quickly as the other children in the class. This was one reason he was so disruptive: he was lost and hated to see the other children forging ahead, leaving him far behind. His poor concentration might also have been associated with feeling switched off from academic tasks, or because he was so connected to digital media that he didn't know how to slow himself down to the pace of the real world.

I wasn't surprised to find he had no behavioural disorder. Even if he had been found to have ADHD or something like it, I *still felt that the amount of TV he watched and computer games he played were a major part of his aggression and poor concentration. I certainly don't believe that computer and video games are evil pastimes to be avoided at all costs, but I do believe they harbour potential dangers; they should be monitored and limited for children. There is a proven link, for example, between regularly playing violent video games and higher levels of aggression in children. Once Brendan had been disconnected, he had a much better chance of learning to focus and regulate his behaviour.*

How, when and why to 'switch off'

Of course, switching off the TV, the games consoles and the Internet connection has an impact on the whole family. It requires parents to be responsible for what can be quite a tough choice. We ourselves may have to give up some TV-watching or Internet-browsing.

We are standing up to be counted when we go against the culture of media and technology saturation in society. Our children may not fully appreciate our decisions but responsible adults have to think beyond the immediate buzz and ease of media to the wider implications for our children and families; if we stay so connected to digital space, we forget to fully inhabit our family space.

The age rating on computer games does not describe the ability level required to play the game; it indicates the development level required to make sense of the game and lessen the likelihood that the player will be negatively influenced by its themes. Despite this, many of us allow our children or young teenagers to play eighteen-rated games. We need to have backbone. If we believe a particular game will be bad for our child, we must say, 'No,' and prevent them playing it. We should not, of course, buy it for them in the first place. If we have strong views about what is good and bad about media, let's talk about them with our families. We can listen to our children's views and help them to understand why we hold ours.

Here are some ideas you may find useful in explaining why you want to reduce or restrict media time:

'I expect that for every hour you watch TV you spend an hour doing something energetic. You only have about six hours from when you come in from school till you go to bed. You have to eat your dinner and do your homework, which leaves about four hours. You can spend half that watching TV or playing computer games and the rest has to be spent outside playing or at least using your brain differently inside, like reading or playing cards.'

'You seem cross that your friends get to watch as much TV as they like. Every family can have different rules and in our family the rule is one hour of TV a day. When you are in your friends' houses you go by their rules. At home you go by ours.'

'Those games promote violence. The whole purpose is to kill people and the graphics are incredibly realistic. I don't believe you'll want to kill someone just because you play that game, but I do believe you'll act more aggressively. As far as I know that is why the game is for sixteens [or eighteens], and that is why it isn't suitable for you because you are still twelve. I don't want you to be aggressive. I like you the way you are.'

'I notice that after you play video games you always seem cross and argumentative. I think it is because you get all fired up by the shooting and fighting [or by the excitement of the racing] and it takes you ages to calm down again. So, unless we can find a good way to burn up the extra energy quickly, the next best option is that you play fewer computer games.'

'Social networking online is fun but you need to balance it with social networking in the real world. Since you got your Facebook account you go out less often to meet your friends and I think that's a bad thing. You can keep using Facebook as long as you keep up your real-world friendships too. I don't want you to live in your bedroom. There are lots of other experiences you need to have growing up.'

The benefits of media-free time

Most families find that by reducing computer and TV time and replacing it with games that can be played as a family, they get along better and feel more relaxed. We parents end up having to invest more of our time in our children and in engaging with them. This is only a good thing.

It can be hard if we remain plagued by near constant whining from our child that 'All of my friends have it and play it,' or 'Nobody else has to turn off after an hour.' We can respond with empathy that it's hard to do something differently from everyone else but ultimately we may fall back on the truism that 'Every family has different rules. These are the rules in our house.' If we stick with our decision consistently, our children will adapt and the whining lessen.

Regularly reassessing the media in our lives

When we want our families to thrive we must live in our families. That is what reducing our exposure to media allows. We must show our children that we accept liability for the choices we make. It's okay to make rules, especially when we know that the rules serve a helpful function. Really we're showing our children that we're prepared to make responsible choices because we accept and acknowledge that they are too young to make them for themselves.

That is not to say that children can never make choices, and the choices we may make now about media will have to be revisited when our children reach their teenage years. Connection to an online life will probably be as important to the social health and wellbeing of our teenagers as being with their friends and others in the real world. But teenagers can take more responsibility and be more accountable for their behaviour.

Keeping communication alive about these issues and discussing the value of the responsibility involved will allow them to grow into their adult responsibility along with their adult independence.

05
THRIVING IN THE THROES OF ADOLESCENCE

Adapting your parenting approach for adolescents

Adolescence is a tricky time for most families to negotiate, never mind thrive in. Many of the parenting approaches that work successfully with younger children seem ineffective, or even cause conflict, during your children's teenage years. Behavioural consequences, for example, lose their power when we discover that we can't enforce the penalties (such as when our teenager storms past us despite being grounded).

Very often, the more we try to control our teenagers the more out of control they become. Adolescence is a time for families to do things differently. The key to this, and maintaining your family's cohesion, lies in understanding what is happening to teenagers and what they need at this time in their lives. It can seem as if everything you knew about being a parent has to be adapted and tweaked as you become the parent of a teenager. However, as long as we remember that we, too, are in a developmental process as a parent, we can grow into our new role as they move towards adulthood.

The search for identity

Identity formation is a central theme of adolescence. Teenagers are trying to work out who they are, what they believe in and where they are going with their lives. Ironically, the route many take is to contradict and challenge the values, beliefs and ideals of their parents. This is not a bad thing, but it can be a big struggle for parents, who feel offended by the, at times, adversarial nature of the challenge. Having those values and expectations in the first place at least gives your sons and daughters some baseline for comparison as they experiment with different styles of clothes, hair, behaviour and attitudes.

It can feel hurtful and rejecting when your son or daughter seems to dismiss your beliefs and ignore your guidance. It can be worrying to see them making mistakes that you know can be avoided. Yet if teenagers don't get to make their mistakes, on the basis of their increasing choices, they may not grow and thrive. It can seem counterintuitive, but sometimes making a mess of things leads to a successful outcome. But this can only happen as long as we remain engaged and connected to help our teenagers make sense of their experiences and learn how to make wiser and healthier choices in the future.

As they struggle to work out who they are, they need us to remain dependably who we are. We can't shift suddenly from being a firm, authoritative parent to their best friend, who just wants to listen to them and never resists them. We need to stand by our principles and our beliefs, and to make some choices on their behalf, if we know that the alternatives are too dangerous for them. We need to remain predictable and secure so that they have their solid base from which to explore and experiment before returning for some care and nurturing.

Identity formation: physical growth

We all know that adolescence is a time of significant physical growth. Most teenagers know what to expect, from hair on their bodies to the development of their sexual organs. Sometimes, though, some of the changes that occur may take them by surprise, whether it is the start of menstruation or having wet dreams. Parents may be embarrassed about talking through these issues so we may try to avoid it, hoping they know more than may be the case. It is worth, at the very least, giving your son or daughter a book about the changes they can expect. Accurate information protects them against the myth and misinformation their peers may be peddling. It's better if you can talk about it, because that leaves the door open for them to check any concerns with you.

And teenagers do worry about their physical changes. Girls who mature early may have a hard time because their body shape makes them different from their peers and brings a different kind of attention from older boys and men. Boys who mature late may be embarrassed by their comparative underdevelopment or feel left behind their peers who have grown bigger and stronger.

Even when teenagers develop at similar times to their peers, they may still worry about how they look and sound, whether they are normal. Adults may downplay or ridicule these anxieties, forgetting about their own teenage years and just how important it felt to be like everyone else. If your body feels wrong to you, then it's easy to believe that others will reject you. This will impact on your self-esteem and may lead to strong mood swings. Therefore understanding and acknowledgement of your teenager's anxieties, followed by reassurance that there are many different kinds of 'normal', may help to smooth their path.

Identity formation: cognitive development

As children move into their teenage years, their thinking becomes more complex. They move from concrete thought to more abstract notions and possibilities. They also develop the ability to reason from a known starting position, coming up with their own new ideas. They can tolerate many competing views, which enables them to improve their debating skills as well as to empathise more keenly.

In practice, this means that their arguments with you will become more reasoned, more logical and, potentially, more challenging as they identify hypocrisies and inconsistencies in your stance on different issues. That is not to say their emotions won't still overwhelm them at times, leading to a meltdown and a dose of irrationality (it happens to us all!), but the potential for reason is greater. They can also grapple with the theoretical and moral aspect of the values we have been teaching and living with them. So, rather than simply accepting that it's good to tell the truth, they can debate the issues and moral complexities of situations in which lying might be an appropriate response (if the truth might hurt).

If we show patience and willingness to engage in debate, teenagers will learn to form mature and considered opinions, beliefs and values to enable them to thrive in your absence.

Identity formation: sexuality

Talking about sex is often a struggle for teenagers and their parents. It is best to start in the pre-teen years, because after puberty has kicked in, most teenagers become shy about their bodies and more reluctant to engage in discussion. But 'the chat' is not a one-off; we need to return regularly to the topic of sex and relationships.

Indeed, helping children to develop a healthy and thriving sexuality involves parents' willingness to engage in moral and value-based discussions about the respect, love, trust, physical and emotional intimacy that are part of thriving sexual relationships. We need to set the context in which teenagers can try to make sense of their feelings, attractions and their energy. Ultimately, they will make their own choices about how they express their sexuality. All we can hope for is that they feel good about it and that it is positive and fulfilling for them.

Identity formation: moral and ethical development

During adolescence, youngsters develop and refine their conscience. A developed conscience enables us to self-regulate our behaviour according to the social and cultural norms we accept. Teenagers need values to determine what is right and wrong. We may struggle to accept that their values are not only influenced by us, but also by their peers, society and the media.

The ability to see ahead, plan and anticipate consequences will guide some of their behaviour, but it may not be fully mature until they are in their early twenties. That is why it's good for them to have some guiding beliefs that can help them to make choices, not simply according to consequences but also to a moral or ethical principle.

If we as parents have struggled to be consistent in the messages we have given our children about what is right, wrong, fair or unjust, they may find it harder to develop a moral compass to guide and direct their behaviour. They are heading for independence and need to understand why they make the choices they do.

Identity formation: becoming independent

The process of separating from your parents and becoming an independent agent, responsible for your actions, begins in toddlerhood and typically continues to early adulthood. In previous generations, independence had occurred by late adolescence, but over the past few decades, the separation from parents has been delayed, with many twenty-somethings still remaining dependent to some degree.

Even though it is natural and healthy for teenagers to withdraw from depending on their parents, we need to remember that they will feel the loss of their previous connection to us. Emotionally and psychologically, independence can be bittersweet. Teenagers may celebrate their freedom, while feeling saddened that their childhood and the ease of irresponsibility is over. All of the different pressures that independence brings, as well as the struggle they may face to wrest that independence from us, contributes to the moodiness that typifies teenagers.

Struggle and conflict in the teenage years

The teenage years are not all about struggle and conflict. Adolescence is a time of rapid growth and development after what may have seemed a comparatively settled and slowly progressive middle childhood. The teenage years are often portrayed as a pitched battle between the opposing forces of stability and maturity (parents) and wildly wanton provocation (teenagers), but it doesn't have to be like this. Engaging with teenagers and being willing to see the world from their perspective can avoid, or reduce the intensity of, many of the conflicts we encounter.

It also helps to remember that teenagers' increasing maturity, creativity and developing insights can be truly stimulating, rather than just provocative. We can take pride in their ability to do more, understand more and achieve more. Teenagers may reject our beliefs, values and guidance, they may betray our trust and create problems for themselves and us, but this is a part of life, so we may have to dust ourselves, or them, off and try again. It is our commitment to, and our love for, our teenagers that will enable them to grow and thrive so that they remain our sons and daughters, if no longer our children.

The role of trust

When your children are small, your consistency, predictability and reliability establish a secure, trustworthy base for them. If they learn that they can trust you, they are more likely to trust other people. However, having a child who can trust others is only half the task; we also need to allow our children to learn to be trustworthy themselves. As you can imagine, this can only be achieved by giving them opportunities to demonstrate their reliability, which means trusting them to do things by themselves or to do things as they have promised to do them.

Planting the seeds of trust early

As we discussed earlier, the sooner we start giving our children small responsibilities with which to demonstrate their trustworthiness, the better. We might give them little jobs, like feeding a pet or wiping a table. Their performance of these tasks, understandably, may show us that they can't be trusted fully. They may not always follow through and they don't necessarily do what they are supposed to.

However, not doing chores properly or forgetting to do them doesn't have major consequences for the family. To be let down in this way is no cause for alarm because we remember that they are children so it is unreasonable to expect them to be reliable all the time. We can accept that they will make mistakes while they are still learning. If we start this process in adolescence, the consequences of our trust being misplaced may be more significant; the situations in which our teenagers find themselves may be more serious (such as choosing whether or not to drink alcohol). We have a higher expectation of a teenager's reliability than a child's so feel more let down if they make mistakes and don't uphold the trust we have placed in them.

Responding when teenagers break trust

When we respond to teenagers who have shown themselves to be untrustworthy, either we can punish them for betraying our trust and letting us (maybe themselves) down, or we can review the mistakes and give them another chance to get it right.

In my experience, fear of punishment should not be the only thing that encourages them to behave well and remain trustworthy. Punishment may lead to a negative spiral of interaction: punisher and punished may develop a negative view of each other. Also, punishing your teenager for untrustworthiness doesn't show them how to be trustworthy the next time. Instead, it may alienate, anger and leave them thinking, 'Why bother trying to be good? They don't trust me anyway.' Furthermore, punishments – consequences – may keep teenagers on a particular track, but only for fear of the consequences of leaving it, rather than because they want to stay on it.

In a truly thriving family, we want to rely on our teenagers to behave well because they know it is an intrinsically good thing that they do. That is why reviewing the situation in which a teenager has betrayed trust, and showing them how to act better next time, will have a more successful long-term outcome. Within the review, we can also highlight instances when our teenagers upheld our trust. By acknowledging the positive aspects of their behaviour, we will encourage our teenagers to repeat it. Trusting others, and trustworthiness, are always demonstrated in our behaviour. As such, we will be more successful if we reinforce positively the trustworthy behaviour that they do show, rather than punishing their untrustworthy behaviour.

Showing our trustworthiness

Creating a secure attachment with our children early in life required us to be trustworthy and responsive. We committed ourselves to being reliable for them, and their ongoing learning about trust means we must continue to show ourselves trustworthy and do as we promise.

Consequently, we must carry the same conviction and behaviour into our dealings with everyone. We are role models to our children when we deal with them directly, but also to other members of our family, friends, business contacts and society in general. Our teenagers watch many, if not all, of these interactions, so we must show ourselves trustworthy in every situation if we are to hope they will emulate our behaviour in their dealings with the world. Teenagers, too, will be quick to point out the hypocrisy in any 'Do as I say, not as I do' situations.

A case in point ...

Gina, aged fourteen, was referred to me by her parents. They were concerned because she had become increasingly oppositional and they found themselves rowing with her about every decision they made that affected her: when she had to go to bed, how much time she had to devote to homework, what she spent her money on and, most recently, her demands to be allowed to go to the local disco.

In my discussions with Gina and her parents, I came to realise that Tom and Annie were very strict with their daughter. Strictness is not a bad thing, but it was apparent that Tom and Annie imposed lots of rules, which were dictated without discussion. It seemed to me that Gina, in her adolescence, was simply starting to challenge the rules and the reasons why they were in place. This was a natural process but shocking to Tom and Annie who, up to that point, had never felt challenged in any way because their word had been law.

Accepting that Gina not only would but needed to challenge them was very hard for Tom and Annie. They had grown up in families where a mother, father or both had ruled with an iron will. As children they had done as they were told, which meant they had grown up as conscientious adults who stuck by the rules and were very dependable.

Tom, interestingly, commented that if he was conscientious it was only because he felt he had to be, not always because he wanted to be. As a consequence he, particularly, carried a lot of resentment about the demands placed on him in work but felt unable to address them with his boss. He and Annie also felt huge anxiety when they had to depend on others as their primary instinct was always to be in control.

I explained to Tom and Annie how important it was to continue to have boundaries in place for Gina to help guide her behaviour but that the time was also right to include her in determining those limits. This was not to say that they should suddenly start to let Gina decide everything that she should do. But if they wanted to be able to trust Gina in adulthood, she had to have the opportunity to learn how to be trustworthy now. Listening to their daughter would reduce her frustration so she would challenge them less.

I used the example of her demands to go to the disco as an area where perhaps they might start to let her expand her horizons while still monitoring and reviewing with her how successfully she could keep her promises. On a practical level, this meant that the three of them had to negotiate the terms under which Tom and Annie would feel reassured enough to let Gina go to *the disco and rely on her to keep herself safe and be ready for collection at the agreed time. This was the focus of one session.*

Understandably, the disco was a source of anxiety for Tom and Annie, who viewed it as a den of teenage iniquity, replete with underage drinking, drug-taking and sexual activity. Like most teenagers, Gina rolled her eyes when she heard her parents voicing these fears. She pointed out that they had to trust her to be responsible and to mind herself.

Indeed, the truth was that she had to learn how to cope with the kind of situations her parents were worried about. Ironically, she could never know how she would react to the excitement, and the potential dangers, until she experienced it. Part of growing into responsibility is being able to practise being responsible.

Ultimately Tom and Annie took the risk and let Gina go to the disco, despite their fears. Gina stuck by every one of the agreed conditions, including being picked up earlier than others. Gina's first involvement in a decision about her proved positive for them all. It was great that she successfully upheld the trust placed in her by her parents. Critically, it gave Tom and Annie the confidence to shift their parenting style away from a dictatorship and to increase the level of autonomy they gave Gina.

In fact, Gina had probably always been trustworthy. Because she had merely been complying with all of their limits (for fear of being punished if she didn't), her trustworthiness hadn't been evident – or it hadn't appeared impressive because her parents had taken it for granted. When she had greater freedom (not total freedom!) to make choices and decisions for herself, with reference to them and their views, it became clear that she was choosing to be trustworthy. This was impressive because it showed she, too, believed trust was important. When she felt her parents trusted her, she had stepped up to the mark.

When and how to protect – and when to step aside

As parents, we can often foresee dangers, dilemmas and disasters on the horizon, depending on what our teenagers are trying to do. We know they might make a mess with the trust we have placed in them because they are still learning to use it.

Sometimes we are best served by letting nature take its course, as long as an outcome isn't too awful. This way, teenagers experience the positive impact of following through on their promises – and the reverse: we may have foreseen the outcome, but 'I told you so …' won't help matters. Rather, we need to make sure they have taken note of the consequences of their actions, and help them to determine whether a different action could, or should, be taken the next time.

We can't protect our children and teenagers from everything – nor should we. The best way for trust to grow and deepen is from trial and error. Even when teenagers have made mistakes and let us down, we need to give them another chance to do it differently.

What to do when tempers flare

Anger is a powerful and at times destructive force within families. It feels like a primitive emotion, giving rise to the release of adrenalin, the 'flight or fight' hormonal response to danger and threat. Most of us experience anger as coming from deep within, almost as though it is central to our being.

Conflict is a natural product of a teenager's attempts to become an individual. It is to be expected that our teenagers will challenge us, our values, rules and behaviour. We can expect some angry outbursts along the way. Our aim is not to eliminate the anger but to help our teenagers regulate it effectively so that they don't act in a way that hurts other people. We can accept that they will be angry at times, just not aggressive.

Understandably, how we respond to them and their anger will have a significant influence on the extent to which it escalates a situation. Just as we may expect them to moderate their behaviour and their language, we too must regulate our own anger, so that we don't become aggressive either.

Keeping cool when the heat is up

Children and teenagers can be incredibly provocative (intentionally or unintentionally) in their behaviour and/or how they speak to us. When we respond angrily, we tend to make bad decisions and say or do things we later regret. At these times we might curse, shout, punish severely or even hit our children.

Research shows that when we are angry, or in conflict with our children or teenagers, they stop focusing on what we say and pay more attention to what we look and sound like; when we become angry, we are less effective at communicating with them.

Regulating our own angry feelings (reducing or containing them), before responding to our children, means that we can approach them more positively, rationally and with a greater likelihood of them hearing what we are saying and resolving the issue at hand. If we remain calm, we show them that it is possible to manage anger effectively.

Managing our anger as parents

The first step to managing, or regulating, anger is recognising it. Regulation acts a bit like the volume control on a stereo. When you notice it's too loud, you turn it down. Similarly, with anger, when you notice it's becoming intense, you reduce it. Understandably, this means that we have to judge first if we are angry, then determine how intense it is. This is harder than it might sound. Many people miss the signs that they are getting angry until they are beyond regulating it.

Being aware of the signs of adrenalin release in our bodies is the best way to spot that we're getting angry. Adrenalin usually leads to physical responses, such as muscle tension, tightness in the chest or more rapid breathing, an increase in heart rate, a dry mouth or butterflies in the stomach. So when we are becoming angry, we may clench our teeth, tense our necks, ball our hands into fists or feel flushed.

As soon as we feel any of these signs, we need to take remedial action. At this point we are still able to think clearly, which gives us the opportunity to do something that will dissipate the adrenalin, enabling us to calm down. If the angry feelings remain unchecked, they will probably continue to increase and intensify, and that is when we may react irrationally or even dangerously.

We need to learn ways to relax if we feel we are growing angry, or use strategies to withdraw from a situation, allowing ourselves time to calm down. Therefore deep breathing – to slow our heart rate and release some of the muscle tension – may prevent an escalation of anger. Walking away may give us the space and freedom to calm ourselves before our anger becomes uncontrollable.

It's helpful to understand what triggers angry feelings and continues to fuel them. Usually the trigger is an event in the here and now, something that has just occurred or is occurring. How angry we get, though, often depends on the experiences that have preceded the event.

Imagine we have a store of anger that has been generated by a number of different upsetting events. It's like a can of petrol: the more upsetting events we experience, the more the can fills. A particular event may trigger us to feel angry, akin to striking a match. When a lit match comes in contact with a petrol can, it causes an explosion. In the same way, a triggering event leads to an explosion of accumulated anger.

For example, if you have a bad day at work, you're likely to bring home your annoyance or frustration. Later, your teenager challenges your insistence that he goes to bed. His refusal might be the trigger, but the power of your angry response may come from the anger you didn't express at work earlier in the day. Your teenager becomes the unwitting, unintended and unjust recipient of a lot of anger that should have been addressed to your boss.

Understanding unresolved anger

Even though their lives have been comparatively short, teenagers may still have experienced enough rejection, criticism, disappointment and bullying (or any number of other hurtful experiences) to have a store of unresolved anger.

Imagine a teenager whose efforts are never seen to be good enough, who always appears to be a disappointment in the eyes of his father. On any given day, that father may criticise his son for not studying, not doing chores to a particular standard or whatever. The son is likely to feel piqued by the disparagement of his work and the dismissal of his effort. He may react with anger that is triggered by this criticism but fuelled by years of such rejection. Unfettered, it could lead to a major row between son and father. If neither is aware of how the criticism has built up to rejection, neither will be able to prevent the inevitable rise of anger and its eventual explosion.

Teenagers can't be expected to be aware enough of their inner world to spot the build-up of their anger without guidance and help from the adults around them. We need the sensitivity and empathy to notice that their feelings may be blocked or 'bottled up'. Then we can redirect them to calm down and help them (later) to express the feelings in words rather than actions. While it may sound straightforward, it can be tricky to achieve.

A case in point ...

Simon was fifteen when his mum, Lisa, brought him to my clinic. She was a single parent and had raised Simon alone. Simon knew who his dad was but had last seen him when he was seven. Until then, his contact with his dad had been sporadic because his dad travelled a lot and had drifted in and out of his son's life.

For the months that his dad was home, he may or may not have made contact with Lisa to see Simon. Naturally this was very disruptive for Simon and Lisa. Lisa eventually gave Simon's dad an ultimatum to either be reliably available for Simon or have nothing to do with him. That was the last time that either Simon or Lisa had seen him.

When he came to see me, Simon was in trouble – in school, at home and in the town. He had been cautioned by the police about an incident in which a slightly older boy's collarbone had been broken during a fight that was supposedly started by Simon. At school, he was considered aggressive and challenging, refusing to acknowledge the authority of the teachers. At home, he had blazing rows with his mother, threatening to hit her on one occasion.

I remember Simon walking into my office with his mother. I sensed his hostility and resistance instantly. Almost as soon as his mother started describing the difficulties she was experiencing, he was calling her 'a dope' and rolling his eyes skyward. At one point he spoke to her quite viciously – 'Shut your fucking mouth! That's a lie!' – as she tried to tell me about a recent row they had had when she had tried to ground him for breaking the TV remote against the wall.

As soon as Lisa left the room, I empathised with Simon. I empathised with how miserable it might be to hear such a string of complaints about yourself and your behaviour. I empathised with how hard he must find school, given that few people there seemed to think positively of him. I empathised with how much work was involved in keeping up a reputation as a 'hard man'. I empathised with how much of a struggle he seemed to have with his mum, which was a shame since she was the person he was closest to.

Throughout all of this Simon sat calmly. As I spoke, he seemed to relax a little, almost as if his hostility was weakening. It may have been that he experienced me as non-threatening or

Stages of anger management

❋ **Identify the things that trigger angry reactions.**
Because we have different tolerances and
personalities, what triggers one person may not
trigger another. When people know what their
flashpoints are, they have a chance either to predict
that their anger is imminent or to avoid becoming
angry by avoiding their triggers.

❋ **Identify the first physical signs of anger rising.**
Become aware of tension, fists clenching, flushing,
etc. The earlier we can notice these signs in
ourselves, or others, the greater the opportunity
to reduce the intensity of the anger or to distract
ourselves from it.

❋ **Learn to regulate the adrenalin that is released
in anger.** Typically, breathing-based relaxation
exercises are most effective. They slow down our

*understanding or on his side. It may have been that he liked the
fact that I seemed to see things from his perspective or that I
seemed not to have judged him based on all the negative stories
I had heard. Empathy is a powerful way of making an initial
therapeutic connection.*

*However, as I continued in my attempts to understand his
perspective on the world, I commented on how sad and hurt
he must feel that his dad had left him when he was seven. He
erupted. He screamed at me, 'It fucking wasn't his fault! That
bitch told him to go! He would never leave me! Don't you fucking
dare blame him!'*

*Suddenly I had a new insight into Simon and how he felt.
Where I had mistakenly assumed that he felt abandoned by
his father, in fact he blamed his mother for the ultimatum she*

heart rates, distract us from the trigger incident
and help to reduce muscle tension.

❁ **Find alternative things to do to defuse conflict.**
Walking away and taking time to calm down works
well in avoiding conflict. Talking to other people
about the triggers for your anger can also help
to decompress the feelings and help you to learn
some practical ways of coping. Talking about your
own feelings ('I feel furious that …'), rather than
blaming someone else, helps to avoid escalating an
argument.

❁ **Process past experiences to avoid building
up an 'anger store'.** This is a longer-term, more
comprehensive anger-management approach. By
dealing therapeutically with past hurts, frustrations,
disappointments, criticisms, rejections, and so on,
we can reduce or eliminate the fuel that causes our
anger to burn intensely and destructively.

had given his dad. This was a crucial insight for the therapy
that followed. The power of his resentment towards his mum,
for what he saw as pushing his dad away, was potent and often
unchecked. Whenever he rowed with her over small points of his
behaviour, it was the anger associated with this resentment that
drove minor rows into major confrontations.

He was furiously angry with her and showed it – not just to
her, but to everyone. I believed that years of hurt and resentment
lay at the root of Simon's anger. It wasn't, however, until these
really difficult feelings had been acknowledged and expressed,
helpfully, that Simon could begin to heal. And he did heal.

It took some time before Simon could acknowledge that his
father had played a role in the events that had occurred. Very
slowly, he came to accept that his dad's failure to see him had

been his dad's choice too. Naturally, this hurt a lot. He was angry with his dad then, especially when he came to see that his dad had abandoned him (whether out of selfishness or unwillingness to challenge Lisa), whether or not his mum had pushed him away. This, too, took time to work through.

Simon and his mum eventually spoke about this in a very emotional session. Lisa had long known that Simon blamed her but didn't know how to get past it and had always justified her actions to him, even though that seemed to make him angrier. For the first time, she accepted that her decision had hurt him. Simon was finally at a point where he could stop blaming his mother. For sure, he still got angry at times – who doesn't? But his anger was no longer fuelled by the years of hurt and resentment so it was less intense and shorter-lived.

Why teenagers get angry

Anger is rarely an entirely random, baseless emotion. However, as was the case with Simon, its source may be misinterpreted or misunderstood. It is usually easy to see the trigger for an angry outburst in a teenager but it requires time, patience and kindness to understand the fuel that keeps it burning. In some situations, at home and in school, it is hard to find the time to explore why teenagers become so angry. What is crucial, however, is the inclination to understand.

It really helps, too, to accept that there are times when our approach to parenting, or our family circumstances, may be provocative to our children and teenagers. We may be willing to accept that we can trigger the outbursts, but are often less willing to acknowledge that we may also contribute to the 'anger store' our children carry. We are not always fair and balanced, or kind and respectful, in our dealings with our children so it is possible that they will grow up with a sense of injustice or hurt.

Research shows that it is our kindness, understanding and concern for children, combined with clear rules and expectations for them, that allows them to flourish. If this has been your teenager's experience of you, then I have no doubt that they're thriving. Even if they come across difficult situations, they will probably have the insight to regulate their emotions, even difficult ones like anger.

Creating healthy social networks online and in real life

Teenagers have always needed, and created, social spaces that are private and separate from adults. Part of their ability to thrive rests on the social networks they create outside their families. This is why they have always congregated in parks, on street corners, in city centres and children's playgrounds. It may seem that they're simply hanging around, waiting for life to happen, but in fact they are developmentally active – flirting, boasting, gossiping, teasing, confessing and discovering that their life experiences are normal.

Think back to your own teenage years: you may remember the comparative innocence of the chat you had with your friends. We spent most of our time ensuring we fitted in. Being part of the group was more important, often, than what the group did. The same is true for teenagers today. Although we may worry that they are less 'innocent', the truth is that their need to hang out, and just be, with other teenagers is a really positive part of their development.

Groups or gangs

Adults often worry about teenage groups, especially when they seem to be loitering, seemingly without purpose. We worry that they will create trouble, either by wantonly destroying or damaging property, or intimidating and persecuting other people. We often differentiate between groups (which we designate as comparatively harmless) and gangs (which have the potential to create havoc). We don't mind groups of teenagers but we fear gangs of them.

It is always possible that teenagers will cause trouble, but so could any other social grouping. The core values and beliefs of any group keep the group together and determine if the group will act pro-socially or anti-socially. If a group of disaffected, angry teenagers feel mistreated by society at large, then they may be a threat. However, the majority of teenagers don't fit this category.

Hanging out online

In recent years, online social networks have met some of the need for teenagers to get together. The most recent research data from the US suggests that 95 per cent of all teenagers aged between twelve and seventeen are now online and that 80 per cent of them use social media sites, such as Facebook and Twitter. If you look at an average sample of what is said and shared on these sites you find the same pattern of 'passing the time' banter, spiced with exactly the same flirting, teasing, boasting, and so on that exists when teenagers gather in real life.

What is different is that their online networks are not private in the same way that our hanging out at the park kept us separate from adults. It is much easier, for example, for parents, other peers and random people browsing on the Internet to observe the communication that passes between them. Also, online social networks can be much broader, with the potential for youngsters to be connected to more social groups beyond their previous potential to have home friends, school friends and sports or social-club friends. While this may be good for expanding teenagers' knowledge, it also means the potential for negative influence is wider.

If we want to continue to influence them, we must educate ourselves about how they use their online social networks and what the benefits and/or dangers are. When it comes to this form of social interaction, though, we may be significantly behind the curve!

Understanding peer pressure

We all worry about teenagers being susceptible to peer pressure. We can sometimes contrive peer pressure to be the experience of a group of 'bad' kids forcing our 'good' child to drink, steal or take drugs against their will. In practice, this kind of coercive peer pressure is the least likely type our children will experience. Most youngsters don't feel forced but, rather, willingly subsume themselves into the culture, values and behaviour of a group of their peers.

But we cannot avoid, or get our teenagers to avoid, peer pressure because teenagers need to be with their peers and they need the approval, companionship and acceptance that friends provide.

The large group exerts a general pressure on its members and tends to dictate their preferences in clothing, music, behaviour, habits and sources of entertainment. The specific friendships your teenager has will be of greater influence than 'group think'. Best friends are the most influential role models for what is acceptable and expected. The subtle pressure to be like their best friends has the most power over your son's or daughter's behaviour.

This is why it helps to take an active interest in your children's friends and to note how they seem to be directing your son or daughter. The dilemma that we face is how much we interfere when that direction is negative. Do we deny access or try to control contact with those friends? Many parents will tell you that too much interference can backfire, and that parental disapproval can strengthen the connection to the very friends you object to.

Ultimately, we have to adopt the premise that 'you can lead a horse to water but you can't make it drink'. Our teenagers have to learn to be responsible with their friendships. We need to observe them closely and monitor their activity. When we have the opportunity to distract them or keep them busy and away from their 'bad' friends, we should take it. But there are times when, no matter what we do, teenagers get stuck with bad company.

A case in point ...

Joan was a divorced mother of three boys. She had split from their dad ten years previously, when her eldest, Patrick, was seven. She was worried about Patrick who, over about ten months, had become exceptionally withdrawn, never leaving the house. He had quit school as soon as he was sixteen. She couldn't understand why he had become so hermit-like because he had had two really close friends and had seemed happy and popular.

He had become very overweight and his GP had just recommended a diet and an exercise routine for him because, with a raised sugar level, he was at risk of diabetes. However, he mostly refused to get off the sofa where he sat all day and played his guitar, the PlayStation or hung out online.

I was very concerned for him because his apparent apathy and laziness indeed had major health implications. Even though he was on Facebook and seemed to be interacting with a wide range of people, he seemed disconnected from the real world. He also seemed to me to be at risk of developing depression. I wondered if he had been struggling with his parents' separation as their divorce had only been finalised the year before and his dad had stopped all contact.

I had no relationship with him and he refused to come and meet me. His mother, clearly, felt unable to motivate him. His dad was entirely absent from his life. Despite this, however, we had to find someone who could inspire him a little to help him realise he had potential and a future. Someone who might persuade him to come and meet me at the very least. The answer came from Facebook.

His mum did a little bit of detective work and identified that Patrick's two previously best friends were still 'friends' with him on Facebook. She knew both of their mothers and approached them, explaining her dilemma. Those mothers spoke to their sons, who were able to explain more about Patrick and his moods than his mother had been aware of. It seemed that for a *while Patrick had been writing online about how much he hated his dad, sounding angry, but that this had dwindled over recent months to the point at which he hardly ever made an appearance online.*

Like a lot of boys, his friends had accepted that Patrick was in a bad space and were waiting for him to come out at the other end. When they heard about how physically withdrawn he had become, they agreed to help out. Shockingly for Patrick, they turned up one evening and plopped down on his sofa. They played PlayStation and hung out for a while, then left. Joan was a bit disappointed as she had hoped this might be a breakthrough moment for Patrick.

However, this was just the beginning of a process. His two friends started calling more regularly, showing through their behaviour that they cared about Patrick. He responded slowly, and Joan heard that he was more active online. Over time, he became more active in life too. He arranged to meet his friends in town one evening, the first outside social engagement he had had in eleven months. I judged this was a good time for his mum to suggest he come and talk to me. He agreed and we began sessions that, as anticipated, were about how let down he felt by his dad's abandonment of him.

Between the sessions and his social interaction, Patrick's life moved outside the limited confines of his home and he became more active and engaged with other people. Having the real-world connection with friends supplemented his online social life and he began to feel a valued and liked member of a group again. Since his two friends remained on board, I asked Joan to persuade them to influence Patrick to fully engage in his life and think about his future.

Online communication and social networking

Online chat, or a series of text messages, makes some elements of communication easier for teenagers. If they are to form their identities fully, they must expose themselves to the world. On the one hand, they are communicating a particular attitude and set of values; on the other they are disclosing intimate details about themselves. These two aspects enable them to validate their opinions and determine the appropriateness of their behaviour and attitudes. But it's hard work and can be embarrassing and humiliating.

Digital communication means they can take time to prepare what they say, so can give a considered response that projects a particular face or attitude to the world. They can counter embarrassment or feeling 'put on the spot' by writing, editing and rewriting their response to what someone has said or asked.

With the extent of social networks and the many hundreds of Facebook friends that most teenagers have, there is also a lot more opportunity for flirting, while being at a remove: they don't have to see the expression on the other person's face if the flirting falls flat or is rejected.

However, this is an inherent problem with online communication too. Without non-verbal reactions, we can sometimes be left in the dark about how someone really feels. Verbal communication, in person, relies heavily on tone of voice, facial expression and eye contact to add emotional meaning to what we say and hear. Emoticons (smiley faces), kisses and acronyms (like LOL: laughing out loud) try to compensate for the emotional barrenness, but they are a poor substitute and most of us follow up with a person-to-person chat if we really want to be sure what someone meant.

It is easy to misinterpret what is communicated in text format, by phone or computer because so much emotional context is missing. Think how much time you have taken to frame certain emails so that someone doesn't accidentally take offence or misunderstand your intention. This may explain a proportion of the falling-outs and rows that occur between teenagers – 22 per cent of whom say that an issue online has led to their friendship breaking down in the real world.

Ensuring safety in social networking

Staying connected with their friends is a vital part of a thriving teenager's life. However, three potentially serious issues can arise in digital communication.

First, despite the considered nature of their responses, or maybe because of it, teenagers can use their phones and the Internet to attack others. Even youngsters who may not think of bullying someone in person can be tempted to join in online (cyberbullying) or to target someone themselves. This type of bullying is made easier by the emotional remove in facing a screen, not the person. Communicating online seems to take away some of our protective social inhibitions. When we don't have to face a person's emotional response to our cutting remarks, for example, we can feel braver and more insulated in being aggressive.

Second, teenagers don't think in the long term about how their behaviour and attitudes, as displayed in their photos and postings online, will be perceived when they are older. Many employers are seeking access to employees', or potential employees', Facebook or social media accounts, and trawl the Internet for additional information about job applicants. Teenagers may think it's okay, within their peer group, to express racist, homophobic or sexist attitudes, but they may be called to account for them later. Many online comments and posts by teenagers during the London riots in 2011 were used to prosecute them for incitement to violence, even if that had not been their intention when they wrote the comments.

Third, there are many predators – men usually but not exclusively – who target girls and boys online to abuse them. Teenagers may not think through the level of exposure that their Facebook page allows. They may believe and trust the bona fides of those who befriend them and disclose information that can make them vulnerable. Even if they are not targeted, youngsters rarely think about the potential recipients of naked or semi-naked photos of themselves that they send to genuine friends, boyfriends or girlfriends. Once information is shared online, you can never take it back. This is a painful lesson that some teenagers learn at great cost.

I don't think that there can be one single recommended approach to how we let children and teenagers engage with the Internet. Given the speed at which media are developing, there are many issues for which we don't have our own moral blueprint. We had no steer from our parents about Internet-related issues because they didn't exist in our childhoods so we must make this up as we go along, basing our approach on our wider value system. Basic rules, taught early, will definitely help.

But given how quickly it is moving, our children and teenagers may have to help us work out what seems best to do. Indeed, use of the Internet could be one area on which we can have truly equal discussions with our teenagers. They may have greater knowledge and experience of it than us so this may be an opportunity for them to feel capable and instructive. However, since most teenagers start their online lives in middle childhood, we, and they, are best served by having some clear rules established before they make their first forays onto the Internet.

* Set a rule about acceptable time limits for being online in any one sitting. (It's really hard to establish the willpower to switch off!)
* Set an absolute nightly cut-off time for all media to make it easier for their brains to wind down to sleep.
* For younger children especially, supervise their time online, so that you can be available to help, direct and instruct. (You can reduce this as they get older, wiser and more clued-in to keeping themselves safe.)
* Use filtering software to minimise or eliminate the likelihood of unwanted pornography being available.
* Set a rule about not clicking on pop-up windows. (These are common portals to pornography and computer viruses.)
* Tell them not, under any circumstances, to share their personal details online.

* Remind older children and teenagers of the potential permanency of any online posts they make.
* Establish an understanding that you will make random parental checks of Internet use and social network use (even if teenagers have the skill to clear their tracks online).
* Pool information as a family, since older children or teenagers may know more than us and can share their experience with their younger siblings.
* Have occasional discussions about the Internet (its benefits and dangers), as a family, to show that you are willing to engage with the issues.
* Set expectations about treating people with the same dignity and respect online as in real life.

Helping teenagers to make good decisions about drugs and alcohol

The best choice for teenagers is to avoid drugs and alcohol altogether. In reality, it is not a choice that many of them make. Research statistics for drug and alcohol use vary significantly across studies and countries, but there is consensus that the majority of teenagers will have tried some kind of illicit drug and alcohol by the time they are seventeen.

The social role-modelling of regular and excessive drinking by many adults means that maintaining a zero-tolerance approach to alcohol rarely works. However, some research suggests that keeping teenagers alcohol free until they are fifteen will significantly reduce the likelihood that they will develop problematic alcohol use in later life.

It is hard to thrive, and stay mindful of the real world, when a substance you have consumed, whether it is a drug or alcohol, alters your mind. As with many other areas of teenage life, we cannot protect our sons and daughters from exposure to drugs and alcohol so our goal is to equip them with the skills to make wise choices.

Factors that influence alcohol use

Teenagers who delay the start of their drinking and learn to drink responsibly are more likely to:

✿ Feel connected, positively, to their family
✿ Have a circle of friends whom they perceive to be supportive
✿ Have a positive attitude to school
✿ Have good social skills that help them withstand some of the peer pressure
✿ Be involved in extracurricular activities, such as sports clubs or youth groups.

Teenagers who drink early and develop a problem are more likely to:

Encouraging responsible attitudes to alcohol

In relation to alcohol, the most important thing we can offer our teenagers is the willingness to talk about it and how it affects people. We need to know and express what alcohol does to our bodies and minds. We need to know and express clearly our values and beliefs about alcohol use. We need to express our expectations about our teenagers' use (or non-use) of alcohol. We need to be willing to listen to, and really hear, our teenagers' views about alcohol.

While I know that teenagers need private space and time with their peers, it is also important that they feel we are aware and concerned about their whereabouts and who they are with. We cannot afford to abdicate responsibility for them when they leave the house, and we must send them off knowing our expectations for their behaviour. It helps them to know the family rules about alcohol use. Unfettered freedom increases their vulnerability to

- ❋ Feel alienated from their family
- ❋ Have experienced parental separation
- ❋ Have a long history of behavioural problems
- ❋ Have problems in school (learning or behavioural issues)
- ❋ Be exposed to high levels of alcohol use in their families (parents or older siblings)
- ❋ Live in a disadvantaged area
- ❋ Have a lot of unsupervised time outside their home.

It may be that all of these factors represent instability within a family and a lack of limits or boundaries on behaviour. This gives teenagers more reasons, more opportunities and fewer obstacles to drinking.

abuse alcohol and, much as they grumble about restrictions such as curfews, they need to know that there are boundaries in place.

How we, as parents and role models, use alcohol remains a critical influencing factor for our sons and daughters and how they may approach it. Alcohol use is one area in which many of us find that we say one thing and do another. We may talk about responsible drinking or abstinence, and still binge drink ourselves. Consuming more than five standard units of alcohol in a sitting is considered binge drinking – that's the equivalent of more than five small glasses of wine or more than two and a half pints of beer. Suddenly our own behaviour can be seen in a different perspective.

We must retain consistency between our expressed views, beliefs and values about alcohol and our own use of it. There are enough pressures and bad examples within society and the media to challenge our desire to promote responsible attitudes to alcohol without adding our own abuse of it.

Promoting safe drinking

When teenagers start drinking regularly, it's like the cork coming out of a champagne bottle: it won't go back in. They are highly unlikely to stop. The focus of our intervention must shift to making sure that teenagers keep themselves and their friends safe. From this point, we need to give them the following messages:

* Drink slowly so that your body has a chance to metabolise the alcohol.
* Count how much you drink so that you can stay within your tolerance.
* Eat before drinking to delay or reduce the drunkenness.
* Drink water between alcoholic drinks.
* Don't drink alone: be in safe company.
* Don't leave friends who are drinking, or drunk, alone.

A case in point ...

Rowan was fourteen when her parents, John and Sylvia, brought her to see me. She was the elder of two children. Her younger brother, aged eleven, had autism and was extremely demanding, regularly leaving the house in turmoil. According to her mum and dad, Rowan, too, was becoming out of control to the point that she had recently been brought home at three o'clock in the morning by the police, incoherently drunk.

This was the culmination of a few months of increasing opposition and defiance in which Rowan had started going out more, ignoring her curfew, and becoming extremely dismissive and disrespectful of her parents. This behaviour was in stark contrast to how she had been during primary school and even her first year of secondary school. She had been a compliant and considerate child and had often been the one to placate or distract her little brother when he was distressed and acting out.

When I explored this further, it seemed that their home tended towards chaos because Bill (their son with autism) was unpredictable and prone to major tantrums in which doors, tables and chairs had all been broken. John and Sylvia admitted that they rarely felt they coped with the challenge of caring for him so dealing with Rowan's insolence and misbehaviour felt like the straw that was breaking the camel's back.

I focused my interest first on what the experience of living at home was like for Rowan. Although she was initially very wary and quite resistant, she opened up and talked once she realised that attendance with me was not about punishment. She described their home as a war zone with everyone on tenterhooks waiting for the next explosion from Bill. She had to keep her bedroom locked and occasionally retreated inside it to avoid getting hurt by him.

She felt that she used to be able to get through to him when he was younger but now she had no clue how to help him. She also resented how much time and attention he took up in the home. 'It has always been about Bill, Bill this and Bill that ... They're forever going to appointments and arguing with the Department of Education about Bill. Nothing is ever about me.'

She felt deeply that she was unimportant in the family. She also had such mixed feelings about Bill, ranging from real sympathy and caring to jealousy and hatred. This seemed like a heady mix to me and really explained why going out, being with her friends and drinking to excess might seem like a solution to the stresses and distresses of being at home.

The horse had definitely bolted, to coin a phrase, with regard to her drinking so it was pointless to try to persuade her to stop. However, in my direct therapy with her, I tried to help Rowan see how her drinking and socialising were an unhealthy way of avoiding her problems at home. I tried to help her to process some of her feelings so that she didn't need to keep acting them out in such a potentially self-destructive way.

I also worked with her mum and dad to try to clarify their values and beliefs about alcohol and to get them to understand *how distressing home life was for Rowan. They were already working to try to deal with Bill's aggression, but they had never really spent any time connecting with Rowan and her experience of Bill and their family life. Understandably, they couldn't just restore calm to the house but they could, and did, let Rowan know that they understood how she felt.*

This was important because it shifted the dynamic between them and Rowan. Prior to this, they had tried to enforce strict rules that she had ignored. After emotionally connecting with Rowan, they were able to talk to her openly about her behaviour and she could hear their genuine concern for her. Rowan didn't stop drinking, or going out, but she seemed to take on a more self-respectful attitude and she did stop coming home drunk. This alone was a relief to her parents, who felt that she would make wiser and safer choices when she was out if she wasn't drunk.

Educating ourselves about drugs

Your teenage son or daughter probably knows more about the different kinds of drugs that are available, and their effects, than you do. It is very hard to influence their attitudes or behaviour when we are less educated than they are or naïve about the topic. There is lots of information available online or from agencies, such as the police or different youth organisations, that we can access to ensure that we don't remain in the dark.

Many schools run drug awareness talks in the evening yet the take-up by parents can be tiny in proportion to the number of children in the school. It is as if we adopt a head-in-the-sand approach, hoping that our teenager either won't come into contact with drugs or that they will be sensible enough to choose not to use them. This will rarely be the case and we need to engage actively with them about drugs.

Drug use: the signs

Sometimes parents have difficulty in identifying that their teenager is using drugs. The following is not an exhaustive list – nor do individual items mean that teenagers are using drugs; in fact, many of these signs, on their own, can be typical of any teenager – but shows some of the behaviour to look out for. We need to be guided a little by our gut feeling that something may be not right. If a pattern emerges of several of these indicators occurring across the three areas, it may be time to take action.

* **Signs in the Home**
  * Loss of interest in family activities
  * Sudden disrespect for family rules
  * Increased lying about activities and whereabouts
  * Finding cigarette rolling papers, pipes, roach clips (like small tweezers), small glass vials, plastic baggies (like very small freezer bags or cling-film bags), remnants of drugs (seeds, etc.)
  * Requests or demands for more money
  * Money or valuables disappearing from home
  * Having more money than you would expect them to have (may be selling drugs to support a habit)
  * Changes in appetite (can be hard to judge because a teenager's appetite varies in accordance with his/her growth and development needs).
* **Signs at school**
  * Sudden drop in school results
  * Loss of interest in learning

- Falling asleep in class or having significantly reduced memory and concentration span
- General defiance of authority and truancy.
* **Physical and emotional signs**
- Shift in friendships and joining a new peer group
- Noticeable change in attitude with big swings in mood or behaviour
- Becoming more argumentative, paranoid, anxious or destructive
- General unhappiness or depression.

How to respond if you suspect drug use in your teenager

It can be incredibly shocking to discover that your son or daughter is using drugs. We can feel helpless or even responsible. Getting some social support for ourselves, by talking with other parents on helplines or in support groups, can alleviate some of the stress we feel. The extra information you gather may also give you better ideas about when you need to intervene.

Begin by letting your teenager know what evidence you have that they are using drugs and asking them to account for it. This is not about proving them to be liars or trying to catch them out, even though they will probably minimise or deny their use. It is about being open, honest and showing yourself to be understanding and focused on solving a problem rather than apportioning blame.

Do let them know how concerned and scared you are and that you only want the best for them. Use your knowledge of drugs to explain what concerns and scares you, and what harm you can see their behaviour causing to them and to the family. Again, don't be too disillusioned if they seem to reject or minimise the risks involved. If they are just trying or experimenting with drugs, a really strong and passionate discussion about drugs, their health and welfare may be enough to dissuade them from further use.

It is likely that your power to control their behaviour is limited now so you must hold them responsible for their own behaviour. This means showing them that they are making choices that may get them into debt, damage their health and disrupt the family. They may also be neglecting their future by not studying. Terrible though it may seem, you cannot rescue them from the harm drug use can cause and they must make the decision to change their behaviour. If they want to do that, you can support them emotionally and in practical ways, such as helping them to break with a particular group of friends or finding other things to occupy their time.

We can still try to put sanctions in place and restrict their contact with certain people, but we have to accept that this may not work. Unless our teenagers have some internal desire to change, our efforts may come to nothing. If the situation worsens and their behaviour seems habitual and/or addictive in nature, we probably need to get direct support for ourselves from a drugs counsellor or a treatment programme. If we can get our teenagers to engage, then drugs counselling or treatment may be the answer for them too.

Making homework and study a part of life, not a constant battle

An area of family life that everyone finds difficult to manage at some stage is homework, study and exams. Frustrated parents, whose children do not want to do their homework or who show no interest in school or state exams, contact me regularly. 'If I don't stand over him he won't do a thing,' is a common enough complaint. Even from early in a child's school career, homework can be a source of major conflict and distress, for both parents and the child. By the time they reach their teenage years, we may feel that the struggle to get them to study is a wasted effort.

Most of us realise, I think, that investing in education gives children greater choice and opportunity in life. Teenagers who put effort into their schoolwork will probably achieve better results, which may lead to third-level college or university. With a third-level qualification, a young adult may have more choice in terms of jobs or careers.

Having been through the school system, and maybe college, most of us can see the long-term benefit of being conscientious about our studies. Even if we never had the opportunity for further education, we can aspire to our children having it, and maybe a more financially comfortable life than we could provide. It's easier to thrive when you have the resources you need – physically, financially, emotionally and psychologically.

Planning ahead

We may have difficulty in engaging our teenagers with this long-term vision when the short-term cost can seem great to them. Why would a teenager want to spend an hour or two labouring over homework, then put an extra hour into revision when they could be chilling out or meeting their mates? Why do homework or apply themselves to study or exams when the payoff seems so far away and intangible? After all, we can't guarantee that working hard at school will give them a better quality of life.

Neurological research has shown that teenagers' brains are immature in the frontal lobes. Practically, this means they are more likely to be impulsive, less able to plan, fail to prioritise effectively and make bad judgements in relation to risks. It is common, therefore, that teenagers have no plan for their future. And this is true of teenagers from all generations – how many people can you remember having a life plan when you were aged thirteen, fifteen or even seventeen?

Until such time that they acquire a life goal that they are striving for, we need to keep the pressure on. How we set up children's homework habits at the start will have some payback in their teen years when they feel they have no choice but to get on with it. Most youngsters get through their first state exams with a lot of external motivation from parents, as well as a sense of obligation. By the time they do their final state exams, they are more likely to have an eye to their own future and, hopefully, the motivation to succeed will have kicked in.

A case in point ...

Mona contacted me, wondering how she could motivate her thirteen-year-old daughter, Rebecca. According to her mum, Rebecca's biggest problem was her attitude. Mona was worried that Rebecca appeared to have no ambition to do well, in stark comparison to her older sister who was a high achiever. When it came to studying, Rebecca typically made statements like, 'I hate geography anyway,' before refusing to open a book.

Mona was very upset by her daughter's apparent rejection of school at such a young age. She came from a farming background and her parents' attitude had been that education was king. There was a very strong work ethic in her family that had been passed down to her and her sisters. Even though she had had farm chores to do, it had been drilled into her that study was the priority. Mona had no recollection of ever questioning this belief and had long ago accepted that education was the key to success. Rebecca's apparent rejection of this had thrown her. She just didn't understand how Rebecca could be so dismissive of school.

When I met Rebecca, I was struck by how unhappy she looked. I thought she was just annoyed at having to come to the session, but as soon as I opened up an opportunity for her to talk, she poured out her distress at how hard she was finding secondary school. She talked about feeling excluded by her peers (she felt they looked down on her), who all seemed to have come into the school with ready-made cliques. She also spoke with some anger about how teachers were regularly commenting to her on how great her sister was and how they expected similar great things from her.

Far from motivating her, the teachers' expectations had simply turned her off school. When we explored why, Rebecca identified *that she was afraid of failing to perform as well as her sister so had decided not to bother competing. When she achieved poor results in class tests, she liked having the excuse that she hadn't put in any effort.*

In school, her difficulty in making friends, and feeling that she didn't fit in, was always on her mind. She hated being reminded of school when her parents asked her about study because she was confronted yet again with her stress over her peers. Peer approval is hugely important, especially for young teens, and not having that approval was distressing for Rebecca. No wonder she snapped every time her mum asked her about school or study.

I acknowledged with Rebecca that the kind of distress she felt could, naturally, lead to a negative attitude. I wondered if it could also be distracting, preventing her focusing on her studies and thinking about her future. Having an immediate worry could easily stop her thinking beyond the resolution of that problem. In that case, it would be impossible to motivate her because she didn't have the emotional and psychological space to think about a plan, never mind working to achieve one.

Rebecca and I shared all of these insights with her mum, who was amazed that her otherwise confident daughter seemed so upset about friendships. Mona took on board Rebecca's sense that she was being compared negatively to her older sister. Even though Mona didn't think that she or her husband actually did compare the two, she realised it was Rebecca's perception of an unfavourable comparison that was important. Mona was concerned about Rebecca's sense that her teachers, too, compared her to her sister and so spoke to the school principal.

I worked with Rebecca and her mum to build Rebecca's self-esteem, to ensure that Rebecca and her mum appreciated her individuality, and to help her feel more confident socially. The concept that achievement is not the only mark of success was important for Mona to acknowledge with her daughter. Rebecca started to thrive again when she no longer felt in competition with her sister and when she became less distracted as her social struggle reduced. She still required a bit of a push to get stuck into study but, importantly, her attitude to school and studying was more positive.

Creating effective homework and study habits

The most effective study habits are developed early, either when children start school or start getting homework. However, even if they haven't been built up over the years, there are things we can do to try to get teenagers focused.

* **Set up a regular homework time.** Try to have a routine in place where your child gets used to doing their homework at a set time. This is easier to achieve when children are younger and can often slip once extracurricular activities begin.
* **Feed them first.** Children and teenagers will be tired and their energy levels may be low by the time they get home, so a snack or an early dinner can really help their concentration.
* **Earlier is usually better than later.** They need energy to stay focused, so it is often more successful to get homework done earlier in the evening.
* **Keep them close by.** With younger children, it's a good idea to sit them at the kitchen table where we are able to keep an eye on them and assist them as necessary. However, as they get older, they may find the kitchen too distracting and a desk in their own room might be the solution.
* **Keep distraction to a minimum.** The kitchen table may not be the best place if your child is easily distracted. You may need to structure the homework time so that other children are occupied elsewhere or that you can be available to keep them focused.
* **Encourage regular breaks.** An adult's attention span is about twenty minutes and a child's can be much shorter

so we must be realistic about how long a child can sit and work without regular breaks. With younger children, you may need to time their work periods for about ten minutes (or shorter if they don't last that long), then give them a short break. The same principle applies to older teenagers studying for exams. Breaking their study periods into twenty-minute blocks can make them more efficient than sitting (their minds wandering) for hours at a time.

* **Make homework a fun challenge rather than a chore.** Sometimes children (especially young children and those with concentration difficulties) like to be challenged to see how fast they can achieve a piece of homework or to see how much of the work they can do in a specified time. If this is the case, simply pull out a stopwatch and make a game of it.

* **Break the homework down to the separate subjects.** The amount of work to be done can also be overwhelming and off-putting for a child. Procrastination can start early, with children avoiding beginning because they feel overwhelmed by the apparent size of the task ahead. Present each part of it separately, by taking out one book at a time rather than piling up all the books needed for the homework.

* **Make study timetables.** With an older teenager, you may need to help them construct a timetable that can show how their course can be broken down and studied in bite-size chunks. Timetabling the work makes it seem achievable and they can have the satisfaction of striking off each chunk of work as it is finished, adding to a sense of progress towards completion.

Effort vs success

The process of doing homework, and even exam study, is more important than what is done. To get our children feeling good about doing their work, we need to acknowledge the effort they put in rather than whether they finished it all or got it all right.

Many professionals tell us that their work is mostly about application rather than inspiration so we need to instil in our children the idea that getting through the grind is as important as feeling good about it. Attempted homework is better than not doing any; having some study under the belt means more might be remembered than if none is done.

Exams: pressures and preparation

Three main factors may be present when teenagers are reluctant to face their exams:

1. They may be anxious about what it will be like (a fear of the unknown).
2. They may fear failure.
3. They may worry that there is too much to do and they have left it too late.

Fear of the unknown can be dealt with by completing mock exam papers. Seeing the layout and structure of the paper and knowing how the papers are marked can help students to feel more prepared. Many schools also run mock exams to familiarise them with the process of being in the exam hall and covering the entire paper in the time allowed.

Fear of failure is best addressed by recalibrating either your or their expectations. Sometimes teenagers have clear goals and put themselves under immense pressure to achieve them. More usually, however, they feel stress from parents and teachers, who remind them of how important the exams are. With all the hype that surrounds state exams, most youngsters are fully aware of what a big deal they are and our additional pressure may be counterproductive.

Breaking the subjects down into manageable study topics may help to reduce the worry of not revising the whole syllabus. In practice, most students have to prioritise the subjects, and topics within subjects, that they will prepare. Hopefully, their teachers will have given them some direction in this regard. Creating and following a study timetable, as mentioned above, comes into its own when they panic about how much there is to do.

Ultimately, we can only take on a support role to try to make the environment and the atmosphere at home as conducive as possible to studying. When the time comes, we cannot sit the exam for our teenagers and they have to want to do well on their own account. If they have the desire to do well, most learn to cope and even to thrive.

Developing a healthy sexuality in an age of Internet pornography

I've already mentioned that sexual development and taking ownership of their sexuality is a central part of adolescent identity formation. Most of us do our best to discuss our views on boy- and girlfriends, how to treat them and what to expect physically, psychologically and emotionally in the relationships our teenagers may form. We see it as an important part of their education and development. We want them to develop healthy and respectful relationships, whether they involve sex or not.

We don't want our youngsters engaging in sexual activity that they are not emotionally ready for. We want them to be comfortable with their own bodies and with the expression of their sexual feelings. We want them to be able to care enough about themselves, and to feel good enough about themselves, to be able to say no to sexual activity if that is what feels best. We, equally, want them to be respectful enough of others not to put pressure on anyone else.

Yet, despite all of our intervention and influence a new, and potentially damaging, source of 'sexual education' exists on the Internet. Pornography of all varieties is so abundant and easily available online that most teenagers cannot avoid being exposed to, and influenced by, graphic sexual images and radically different values from those we may intend to pass on.

Filtering the media messages

We are aware enough of the real world in which we live to understand that we are not the only people influencing and offering guidance to our youngsters. We are well aware that their peers have strong views and lots of information (some accurate, some not). We also know that TV programmes and magazine features contain sexual images or themes, which also have an impact on our children.

Once we are aware of the other influences to which our children are exposed, we can address them and either let our views coincide with what they teach or contradict them. If we know, for example, that our child watched a programme that addressed homosexuality, we can discuss our views on the subject. If a movie featured or referred to rape, we can talk about what that means and how it contradicts our values.

Pornography has been around for generations and may well have featured in our own nascent understanding of sex. However, I can almost guarantee that the extent of our children's and teenagers' experiences and exposure to it will dwarf our own. They are growing up with an Internet that offers them almost unlimited access to vast amounts of pornography of every type.

Being aware of Internet pornography

Even if they don't go looking for it, our teenagers can be exposed to pornography unexpectedly, through pop-up links and websites that are retrieved by search engines in response to innocuous word searches.

Recent research estimates that 12 per cent of our five- to seven-year-olds and 16 per cent of eight- to seventeen-year-olds have unintentionally clicked on a link to pornography. In truth, reliable and consistent data about the amount of pornography available, and its consumption by children and teenagers, is difficult to come by. Some estimates suggest that there are between 250 million and 420 million discrete pages of pornography on the Internet and that about 25 per cent of all Internet searches are for pornography.

Other research suggests that two out of every five older teenagers admit to seeking out such sites. Distressingly, what they find is far more explicit and wide-ranging than the 'top shelf' magazines available to earlier generations of teenagers.

Internet pornography and addiction

Physiological addiction may occur with pornography. Graphic and highly sexual images and videos invariably pose women in erotic positions so that the viewing male is aroused quickly and instinctively. Feel-good hormones flood the brain and then, typically, the sexual rush is copper-fastened by the climax of ejaculation. Instinct overcomes rational thought with men's natural sexual drive ending in overdrive. The physiological high is intrinsically rewarding for men and boys so, understandably, they return for more of the same. Troublingly, this can mean hours of skimming pictures and videos, with an ever-increasing desire for more, and different, sexual arousal.

Ultimately, the images become less satisfying than they were when viewed initially, refuelling the constant search for 'better', more arousing pornography. This is the mechanism by which men and teenage boys may begin to search out every fetish, perversion and sexual experience online. They may consume bestiality, bondage, rape, sexual torture and even child pornography in their addictive desire to reach an ever more elusive sexual arousal.

The impact of pornography addiction on relationships

Research evidence suggests that pornography addiction of this kind leads men to become dissatisfied with their relationships. Women in the real world cannot attain the stylised ideals portrayed in pornography, which typically portrays women as objects and commodities to be used, not people to be related to. Men begin to dissociate emotional and physical intimacy, which together are at the heart of successful, committed, long-term relationships.

With their sexual appetites jaded and their sexual expectations skewed, men find their real sexual relationships unsatisfying. Thus isolation and disconnection can develop. This is equally problematic for teenage boys, who have to cope with a range of adolescent issues, such as spots, extreme self-centredness, bodily changes, peer pressure and shyness. With an easy supply of nudity and sex on demand, it is no wonder that a teenager will choose arousal and repeated masturbation to escape from the real world of teenage strife.

The impact of pornography on sexual development

For younger teenagers and children who repeatedly view pornography, there is also the danger that their sexual development will be distorted by the images they view. Pornography objectifies sexuality. It makes violent sex seem normal or commonplace. It creates the belief in youngsters that sex is external and that they don't have to give of themselves emotionally to participate. They can be affected for ever by the images they see.

Once witnessed, sexual acts and images are not forgotten. They are stored and will create the context from which children will eventually try to make sense of, and process, their real-life experiences. If that context is skewed, unbalanced and unreal, they may grow up to have no moral or value compass by which to make good and healthy sexual decisions in later years. They may be confused, dissatisfied and unable to form healthy sexual relationships.

A case in point ...

Brian, aged twelve, was brought to me by his parents, Michael and Suzie. He had broken down in tears one night, describing how he and an eleven-year-old boy who lived near them had been 'doing sex stuff' for the previous eight months. He told them he was ashamed of his behaviour and that he felt so guilty he sometimes wished he were dead. Needless to say, Michael and Suzie were very upset and terrified at the thought that Brian might kill himself.

I established, early on, that the other boy involved was already attending the Child and Adolescent Mental Health Service and had been attending an equivalent service in the UK for a number of years. Apparently there were many concerns about his behaviour, including sexualised acting out, which had been identified in the UK prior to the family moving to Brian's estate the previous year. This discovery had done little to quell Brian's parents' anxieties about their son and what had happened.

Brian seemed really embarrassed as he gave me a very matter-of-fact account of the kinds of things he had been doing with the other boy, Dan. It had started when Dan had invited Brian up to his room and, after they'd looked at various innocuous YouTube clips of TV bloopers, he had asked Brian if he could keep a secret. When Brian said he could, Dan clicked on to a clip from a website of a man and a woman having oral sex. Brian recalled being amazed and unable to look away from the screen before Dan went on to click through to several other videos.

Nothing else happened that day but, on subsequent visits, Dan and Brian had watched more pornography before Dan had dared Brian to try out some of what they were watching. Dan offered to kiss Brian's penis and Brian, slightly embarrassed, had agreed. So began months of secret meetings, lots of sexual touching, mutual masturbation and oral sex. All the time, their *activity was preceded by sessions of watching pornography. 'It was like we were trying to out-gross the other with the sick stuff we would find,' explained Brian, at a later session.*

Michael and Suzie seemed naïve in their understanding of Brian's behaviour and admitted that they had never talked to Brian about sex as it hadn't seemed relevant. Their own discomfort at discussing sexual activity was clear from my meetings with them. It was a big challenge for them to talk to Brian, but it was vital for them to normalise discussions about sex and to become more open and comfortable when talking about it. I strongly encouraged them to talk outside the sessions with Brian about his activities and about what he had seen online.

There was no denying that the sexual activity that Brian had experienced, with no other context than a foundation of explicit pornography, had been mind-blowing for him. His risk of suicide turned out to be minimal because talking to his parents that first day had been like bursting a balloon: the pressure of the guilt, secrecy and shame had dissipated significantly.

Nonetheless, he and his parents needed to be mindful of the messages he had picked up and, where necessary, his parents had to challenge and counteract his perceptions of what was 'normal'. While I was able to empathise with the stress, embarrassment and shame that Brian felt, I didn't want him to receive my value messages about what I believed was okay or not okay. He needed to hear, from his parents, what they believed.

He also, crucially, needed to hear their views while knowing that they loved him and could accept him and his behaviour. To ensure greater openness and proper communication, it was vital that they showed him they wanted to engage with him about this sexual life he had hidden from them and felt guilty about. They needed to help him discuss things such as homosexuality – what it meant for them and what it might mean for him – and to understand that sexual exploration at his age did not define his developing sexuality.

They needed to help him understand the context for what had happened. He needed to see his own behaviour and experience as a real part of his life, but not as the only part of it. Brian had many years of sexual development and exploration ahead of him. To me, preparing his parents for this, by helping them create a clearly formed family perspective about sex and sexuality, seemed as important as preparing Brian.

The importance of discussing sex in the context of relationships

Most of us will attempt some form of sex education with our children and teenagers, but the one-off 'chat' is rarely sufficient. Sex education needs to be an ongoing process and it must highlight the interpersonal nature of sex and place it firmly in the context of relationships.

We must explain sex, emphatically, as shared intimacy between equals; care and consideration should receive the same billing as biology. When our children have a clear sense of our moral and value base for sexual relationships, they have a reference point for the pornographic images and clips they will see. Simply trying to block the pornographic world from our children and teenagers is unlikely to be successful because the opportunities they have for accessing it online will become increasingly hard to patrol. Also, like every other area of parenting, we cannot fully protect our children from harm so we need to give them the coping skills to ensure they can avoid it or cope when it comes their way.

Unpalatable though it may seem, we need to talk about pornography with our children from the age of about thirteen. Our options include trying to get them to think critically about the pornography they have either seen or will see. Teenagers engage with moral dilemmas like the social and political mores that pornography displays or how pleasure can be derived (or not) from others' pain.

We will probably go to and fro with the issue of pornography and its impact on, or relevance to, our teenagers as their world expands beyond our immediate reach and our desire to protect or control. As each of our children grows and develops, we will be refining, and at times re-evaluating, our beliefs about healthy sexual development and respectful physical and emotional intimacy.

Importantly, we cannot afford to be blinded to the reality that the world of pornography is out there and that our children will engage with it at some level. By giving them a core sense of respect for themselves and for others, we can strengthen their resistance to the social and sexual messages that threaten to sexualise them in particular ways, and to those that just confuse them. Ideally, we will have given them a rationale for why it is good to resist, or at least be critical of, the messages that pornography implicitly gives.

06
THRIVING UNDER ADVERSITY

Developing the skills for unexpected change

It would be nice to think that life will always progress smoothly for our families, but it rarely does. We are regularly confronted by situations that we have never faced before. Sometimes we cope well, but at others those changes can be shocking, distressing and overwhelming. At such times, we may feel as though we will never thrive again.

As long as we feel we can cope with these challenges, they help us to grow and develop. Learning to deal with new situations develops fresh skills, greater maturity, and can help us become more confident and strengthen our character. However, when we don't feel we're coping, they threaten to destabilise our families, leaving us doubting ourselves; they may also damage our self-esteem and the very fabric of who we are.

We need challenges to keep us forward-moving and thriving. Without challenge, we're likely to remain stagnant and stunted in many areas of our physical, emotional or psychological lives. As with many areas of growth, however, the ideal situation is to have balance. We need enough of a challenge to feel motivated to learn, develop and achieve, but not so much that we feel overwhelmed and unable to cope or move forward. Similarly, we don't want too little challenge; then we don't bother to strive for new understanding or personal growth.

Life challenges are, generally, emotionally stressful. A little emotional stress can be good because it keeps us alert, focused and emotionally energised. If that stress builds too much, though, it may inhibit our performance to the point that we stop coping and may even cause us to regress psychologically or emotionally. Learning to understand, regulate and process our emotions is the most protective thing we can do to manage the emotional stresses that adversity will bring.

The impact of life change on stress

In Chapter 2, I spoke of how routine is beneficial to small children and how, when their routine changes, they may be distressed because they are faced with unpredictability. They don't yet know how the new routine will operate so they can't determine if they will be okay. Unpredictability in life causes anxiety.

It's the same for adults. When we are faced with change in life, we are thrown out of our comfort zone and must adapt to the new circumstances. We can suffer from the same stress and anxiety of 'not knowing'. We may worry about what will happen, and whether or not we will cope. Moving to a new set of circumstances means losing the old set; we may miss them, and grieve the loss. We may be angry about or resistant to the change, too, if we feel it has been foisted upon us, is unfair or overwhelming. We experience the sadness, anger, instability and worry we feel about change as stress.

Sometimes, when we have decided to make the change, we can mitigate some of these feelings, because we feel more in control or more prepared for it. When the changing circumstances are outside our control – when they are not our decision – we are often more resistant to them, adding to our stress.

Understanding what determines emotional health and wellbeing

Real emotional wellbeing requires us to recognise and respond consciously to our own emotions, regulating them so that we remain thoughtful and determined in our behaviour, rather than simply reacting to our feelings.

The first step is to be aware of what we're feeling as we're feeling it. Can you spot the signs that you're getting angry? If you can, are you able to describe the extent of your anger (irritated, frustrated, annoyed, angry, furious, and so on)? Most importantly, can you tell someone else about your anger, or reduce its intensity, rather than show him or her by having the equivalent of a tantrum? My guess is that, like most people, sometimes you can and sometimes you can't.

Our prevailing mood and life history will be determining factors in how successfully we can manage our emotions at any given moment. If we are already stressed or angry, we are less likely to be able to regulate any additional annoyance generated by someone's actions. If we grew up in a family where anger was regularly acted out with screaming or violence, we are less likely to be able to regulate anger triggered by present circumstances.

How effectively we have learned to understand and deal with feelings will influence how we respond in the here and now to emotive issues. When we have never dealt with past emotional 'baggage' we can find that troubling feelings will regularly re-emerge and may trip us up, keeping us stuck in old, unsuccessful, patterns of behaviour.

A feeling (of some kind) precedes all behaviour, and most behaviour is simply a response to the feeling. By tuning in to our feelings, and being able to regulate how we experience them, we can learn to regulate and control our behaviour more effectively.

Regulating children's feelings

Hopefully, as we have grown up, we have been helped to learn about our feelings, recognising what they are and being able to determine the intensity with which we feel them. This is a job that your parents did for you in the first instance. Hopefully, they spotted when you got upset and tried to offer understanding and comfort to soothe you. So, assuming we have learned to recognise and regulate our own feelings, we can tune in to the feelings of others. We notice when our children feel upset, angry, sad, disappointed, scared, happy ,and so on. We don't expect small children to stop crying without assistance from us. Instinctively, we try to respond to such situations with understanding or sympathy, helping them to feel less upset.

As children get older, we expect them to regulate their own feelings, but unless we have shown them how to do this, they are likely to struggle. We know, too, that their feelings will partly determine their subsequent behaviour. A child who struggles with expressing difficult feelings may show them in difficult or challenging behaviour. For example, a child who is feeling angry may slam a door. A child who is anxious at our leaving may run after us, crying intensely. A child who feels jealous of his sister may pinch her. When behaviour is considered 'bold', it often impedes our emotional response to the underlying feeling. We end up angry about the child's behaviour and tend to reprimand them without thinking about, or trying to deal with, how they feel.

These are lost opportunities because I can guarantee that when children feel differently they act differently too. If we respond in an emotionally supportive way, we can powerfully influence children's behaviour. When we can understand and acknowledge their feelings, they don't need to keep showing them to us in misbehaviour.

The role of emotional support in changing children's behaviour

Let's start with empathy, the ability to acknowledge somebody's feeling even if you don't share it. When we empathise with children, they experience congruence (a good fit) between their feelings and the current events or circumstances. When feelings and experience fit, we can process and deal with them. When feelings are at odds with experience, we may find ourselves stuck with the feeling.

Imagine that a nine-year-old girl comes second in a running race she hoped and expected to win. At the end of the race, she is likely to be crying or upset, maybe even angry about losing. One possible parental response, to cover embarrassment at the tears, may be, 'Shush, you're a big girl now, stop crying, you're fine. Sure didn't you come second? That's great.' In this instance, there is a mismatch between the girl's experience, her disappointment, because winning the race was important to her, and what she is told by her parent ('You're fine, you did great anyway'). She is now stuck with the feeling of disappointment and is unable to process it. She will probably remain sad, or angry, and moping for ages.

Imagine the same scenario but this time the parent tries to be emotionally supportive: 'You seem so disappointed. After all your preparation and hard work, you didn't win. No wonder you're sad.' In that moment, she experiences emotional congruence, a fit between her experience of being disappointed and being told by her parent, 'You seem so disappointed.' She can now truly feel the hurt of disappointment, because the experience has been validated by the adult's empathetic response. She will probably cry louder for a minute or so, then quieten and get on with the rest of the day, perhaps preparing for another race.

In truth, the girl's disappointment in each scenario retains the same level of hurt, but in the first scenario the sadness and disappointment linger; in the second, they pass quickly. The disappointment is dealt with when she experiences emotional congruence as a result of the adult's empathy.

'Unblocking' stuck feelings

If we don't empathise with children, they don't learn to deal with their feelings. When feelings are particularly troubling or painful, as may be the case when families suffer adversity, their most likely response will be to ignore or block down the feeling. Many of us use the phrase 'bottling it up' to describe how we can store feelings in some hidden location within ourselves, denying – or at least ignoring – their presence.

We can distract ourselves from our feelings in many positive ways. In the short term, this may be a healthy or protective coping strategy if the feelings are very powerful and threaten to overwhelm us (like a child's grief if their parent dies). Children and teenagers may turn to music, friends or sport to keep themselves busy and occupied so that they don't have time to feel the painful emotions.

In the longer term, those feelings remain stored up and may sometimes be unleashed by a specific event. With a bereaved child, a news report might refer to a car accident in which a parent is killed; this may lead to an unexpected eruption of their own grief. Over time, we may have accumulated a large store of unprocessed feelings that may merge into a single feeling of anger.

If we store lots of feelings we will find it harder and harder to keep ourselves distracted from them. Worryingly, many children, teenagers and adults turn to negative outlets, such as aggression, violence, self-harm, withdrawal and eating disorders, to stay dissociated from the real feelings inside us. Teenagers and adults may use drugs, alcohol, pornography or gambling as unhealthy ways of dissociating. Many addictions can be understood as behaviour people use to avoid dealing with the real world and the pain of their real-world experiences.

Thriving when the going gets tough

In the rest of this chapter, I have identified six common adverse situations that families can experience. In each, remember that every family member, while experiencing the same event, may have his or her own perception of and emotional response to it.

Unless families have the opportunity and skill to be emotionally supportive of each other, there is a danger that strong feelings may be repressed or bottled up. It this occurs, new and challenging behaviour may emerge, typified by anger and aggression, which may threaten the stability and the ability of the family to thrive.

Thriving families have parents who make an effort to tune into their own and their family's feelings, especially in the face of adversity, when we will be more considerate, thoughtful and understanding; we will be able to think beyond the fact that someone is behaving badly and to consider why. Rather than responding to the behaviour in isolation, we can try to respond to the feeling empathetically.

This enables children to feel and understand their emotions, making it more likely that they will deal with and process them. Difficult or challenging behaviour doesn't emerge nearly as much in emotionally attuned families, who cope well with adverse life circumstances. It is not that they don't have strong or difficult feelings, they just deal with them effectively.

Protecting your children from the risk of being bullied

Bullying is the insidious, repeated and intentional harassment of someone and is endemic in society. We have all experienced it either first hand or as witnesses. While we may expect it in childhood, particularly in schools, it is present in all social groups and at all ages. We are aware that it exists but, curiously, it is not always challenged.

Bullying typically involves an imbalance of power in which the aggressor lacks empathy or concern for their target. Indeed, some bullies have contempt for their victim, which makes it difficult for the target to solve the problem themselves. Often, they recognise that they don't have the strength to stand up to the bully alone because it is clear to them that he or she has a lot of power.

When children, especially, are targeted in this way, they need others to stand up for them and help to stop the bullying. More often than not, this needs to be adults who can regulate and contain the behaviour of the bully. Most often it is 'nice' children who get picked on; children who are polite, sensitive, biddable and nervous

The bystander in bullying

Research shows that when bystanders feel empowered to oppose bullying, or to tell an authority figure about it, bullying rates drop. In most instances, though, they feel neither able nor willing to step forward. There are four typical reasons why bystanders don't get involved.

* They are afraid of getting hurt.
* They are afraid of becoming a new target for the bully.
* They are afraid their intervention might make the situation worse.
* They don't know what to do to help.

When you talk to children about their experience of seeing other children picked on, we discover that their decision not to get involved is often a tacit acceptance of the bullying, or the prevailing culture and attitude

may be targeted because they lack a 'hard edge' and don't want to offend anyone by appearing rude or aggressive, and are unwilling or unable to retaliate.

The nature of bullying

Bullying can take many forms. Typically, however, it falls into one of three categories. It may be physical (violent aggression, pushing, tripping), verbal (name-calling, teasing, taunting, racist or homophobic abuse) or psychological (exclusion, humiliation, isolation, threats). The purpose is always the same: to try to exert greater power at the expense of others.

'Cyberbullying' describes bullying that occurs digitally or online. It can include verbal bullying through text messages, instant messaging that permits bullying to occur. The kind of response that some children give as to why they don't get involved includes:

* The bully is my friend.
* The kid being bullied is not my friend.
* He isn't standing up for himself so why should I bother standing up for him?
* She's weak and a bit of a loser.
* It's not worth being called a 'rat' or a 'squealer' to tell anyone else about it.
* It's just too much hassle.
* I'm better off on the inside than the outside of the group.

While these responses show the sometimes invidious position that bystanders can be in, they also demonstrate that most youngsters' priority is to mind themselves; reaching out to the target is hard.

online or on social networks. Similarly, exclusion, threatening and humiliation can also occur in any of these digital forms.

Signs of bullying

It can help to notice if your child is being bullied because they often feel unable to tell you. They may think that parents' intervention will make the bullying worse, or they don't want to upset or worry you. It may be that they feel so worn down that they believe telling you won't, or can't, make a difference or they may fear we will criticise them for not coping.

To counteract their reluctance, we need to adopt a habit of checking in with our children and being prepared to step in and speak up for them. Bullying may be physical, behavioural or emotional.

* **Physical signs include:**
  * Unexplained cuts, bruises or other marks on the child's body.
* **Behavioural signs include:**
  * Unwillingness to go to school
  * Withdrawal from clubs or activities
  * Attention-seeking (causing rows or fights at home, niggling at siblings)
  * Changes in friends and who is calling to the house
  * Poor concentration in school
  * Falling school performance
  * Increased requests for pocket money or an increased number of things 'getting lost'.
* **Emotional signs include:**
  * Unexplained mood swings
  * Becoming withdrawn and seeming isolated at home
  * Visible anxiety or distress at school times or related to friends
  * Becoming clingy.

This list is not exhaustive, and the presence of any of these signs may not necessarily mean that your child is being bullied. However, if several such tell-tale signals are present, it is definitely worth exploring them with your child.

A case in point ...

Paul was fifteen when his parents brought him to me because he had become isolated and withdrawn. He rarely went out to meet his friends, had dropped out of all sports and regularly complained of being sick and unable to go to school. Worryingly for them, he refused to talk to them and denied any problems. He was due to sit his Junior Certificate exam that year and his parents felt that he had become increasingly depressed since the end of the previous school year.

When I met with Paul, he did indeed seem depressed and very withdrawn. He sat very quietly while his parents spoke to me and I anticipated that it might be quite hard to develop a rapport with him. However, as soon as his parents left the room, it was as if a dam had burst; he spoke fluently and passionately about his life.

He had little enthusiasm for anything. He was listless and lethargic at home. He saw no future for himself. He was argumentative and dismissive with his parents. He also confided to me that he had thought about suicide but had never taken action or made specific plans about how he might do it.

Things had clearly reached quite a serious stage for Paul. He identified the start of his troubles as an incident on the rugby pitch during a schools' friendly, in which his shorts were accidentally pulled down in a tackle, exposing his bottom. This had happened around Christmas of the previous academic year. Since then, he had suffered homosexual taunting, with some lads blowing kisses, commenting about his 'sweet little arse' and generally ridiculing him.

He had been in several fights, responding to the provocation with his fists but it had made no difference. If anything, the problem had escalated. When school had finished for the summer, the taunts had continued online, so that when he had returned to school in September, he had had no respite and no refuge. Remarkably, he had never said anything about it to his parents. He admitted to feeling relief at having shared all these thoughts and feelings with me.

It seemed to me that his changes in demeanour, behaviour and mood were all attributable to the bullying he was receiving in school. No matter what he did, he continued to be targeted. This was a situation that required intervention from his school. The first step was to tell his parents.

Paul was really anxious about telling his parents. He believed that his dad would be disappointed in him that he seemed so weak. He was afraid that his mother would overreact and make approaches to the parents of the other boys, exposing him to what he believed would be further ridicule for having his mum fight his battles for him. When we did speak to them, therefore, we highlighted his worries so that his parents could understand them and respond to them.

As it turned out, they were shocked that he had been so upset and carried so much hurt for so long. It explained, for them, the nature and extent of his emotional stress and withdrawal. They went with Paul to speak to the principal of the school, who did not try to deny the potential for bullying there. He accepted that there was a problem and intervened to stop it.

While the bullying stopped after the principal had spoken to the boys involved and their parents, it took Paul some time before he began to believe that things would stay changed. He remained wary of the other lads who had picked on him. We worked on rebuilding his self-esteem and getting him involved again socially and in sports – though rugby proved elusive: he never felt confident that he would be fully included in the teams. However, he started to play soccer with the school team and made new friends through that. As expected, when he felt reconnected with his peers, his mood improved and he started to believe in himself more.

Who bullies?

There is no typical profile of a bully. Sometimes we can assume that they have low self-esteem so bully others to hide their insecurity and make themselves feel important. However, research shows that bullies usually have average or above average self-esteem. They do have problems with aggression and empathy, though. Bullies do not consider the needs or feelings of those they target. They have learned to exert power by

coercive methods and have an aggressive temperament
that was not regulated by their parents. Children
who bully need to learn about empathy and realise
the impact of their behaviour. They need to learn to
control and manage their aggression.

Supporting the bullied child

If our child comes to us with the news they are being bullied, our first
instinct is often to spring into action – fast. But it is important that
we recognise this instinct, and take a step back from it. The single
most important thing you can do in this situation is listen. In the
first instance, your child may not want you to intervene; they may
just want you to understand the struggles they are having. Ironically,
we have to be careful not to overprotect our children. Sometimes if
we have been their 'thick skin', trying to protect them from all harm,
we may have unintentionally denied them the opportunity to learn
the skills to protect themselves.

Once they feel understood, you can help them to develop self-
protective skills by building their self-esteem (see Chapter 4) and by
teaching them to be assertive. Sometimes it's enough to equip your
child with the skills they need to address the bullying themselves.

Assertiveness can include making and holding eye contact,
saying no clearly and loudly, and standing tall in their physical
posture. You can also teach them phrases or responses to taunts or
teasing that are assertive but not aggressive. Ignoring taunts rarely
stops bullying. Most bullies increase their taunts until they can see,
from their target's response, that they have succeeded in hurting
their feelings. We can encourage our children to show outwardly, at
least, that they don't care what is being said about them by making
a response that doesn't indicate hurt or upset. Children may like to
imagine that they have a slippery invisible shield around them that
cruel words cannot stick to. Here are some examples of assertive
verbal responses:

Cyberbullying

This is a relatively recent phenomenon so I have included some tips for understanding and dealing with it that may differ from, or be in addition to, the responses you may make to bullying in other environments. Do remember that one-off comments on a social networking site or in a text message may be nasty and hurtful, but unless they are repeated or sustained they don't necessarily constitute bullying.

✻ Online harassment can often be perceived to be more remote, impersonal or anonymous so is often perpetrated by youngsters who wouldn't ordinarily be aggressive or bullying.

✻ Sometimes the identity of the aggressor can be masked online or with barred or hidden mobile numbers; a target may not know where the bullying is coming from.

'Yes I have red hair, good that you noticed.'
'Yes, I am short, like lots of the population.'
'No, I'm not gay, but happy people are fun to be around.'
'That may be your opinion, but I don't agree.'
'It's amazing, but I can see better with my glasses on.'
'Gayness seems to be on your mind a lot.'
'You can slag me all you want but I know I'm a good person.'

If a child can repeat the taunt, it shows they have heard it. This is more powerful than simply ignoring it. If they can repeat a taunt and maintain eye contact, showing themselves to be unafraid and unfazed by it, many bullies will move on to pick a different target. They are more likely to seek out a child who is distressed by their taunts.

Do notice if things seem to continue or get worse because then you may have to intervene directly with the other parents or the

- ❉ Youngsters may feel less responsible for their online behaviour because there are few or no consequences for what they do online.
- ❉ Online bullying often extends the reach of bullies out of school and into the home of the target.
- ❉ Online taunts spread quickly and targets may feel they have no refuge or relief from the stress.
- ❉ In response, keep screen grabs of social networking pages and keep texts but don't reply or engage in online or text 'chat' or mutual taunting; it indicates clearly to the bully that they are hurting their target.
- ❉ Report, with evidence, the kinds of online commentary that your child has received to the school (if the perpetrators are fellow pupils) or clubs (if they are affiliated to any) or in extreme circumstances to the police.

school to ensure that the bullying is stopped. Time, with support from you and their friends, can help them to recover their self-esteem and self-confidence.

Keeping families strong in parental separation

When parents separate, it changes the structure of a family. The breakdown of the two-parent unit means that everyone in the family has a lot of adjustment to make. Without care, respect and mindfulness of the impact, parental break-up can destroy family functioning and create a legacy of mistrust, hurt and loss that can pervade the relationships children form in adulthood.

Planned separation: telling the children

In an ideal world, parents will sit down with their children and explain about their joint decision to separate. They will be able to agree that separation is the best option to meet their individual needs and, consequently, that it will be better for the family in the long run. In many cases, parents are not in agreement about the reasons for their separation – or even the need for it – so their children may receive mixed and confusing messages.

When parents split up, it is typically because the level of conflict has become so great that the parents cannot put up with it. In other situations, the required level of trust has evaporated. Alcoholism, gambling, affairs and a range of other behaviours may underlie the increase in conflict or the breakdown in trust. Sometimes the separation occurs by mutual consent; more often it is pushed for by one parent.

It is easy for a parent to feel angry about the breakdown and to blame their partner for the split – 'I don't want to leave, this is your mother's idea'; 'We wouldn't be separated except that your dad wanted to go and live with her' – but blaming or criticising your partner jeopardises your child's relationship with that parent. It may also weaken your relationship with your child if they feel protective of the other parent. Unless the other parent is abusive, your child will benefit from a positive relationship with them. Maintaining a good relationship with both parents, especially after a separation, is central to his or her ongoing healthy development.

There are some helpful dos and don'ts to consider when telling children about separation:

* Do make sure that you both give the same message about why you are separating.
* Do try to be as honest as possible about why you are separating.
* Do allow and encourage children to express their feelings and to ask questions.
* Do acknowledge that their feelings may seem complex, upsetting and hurtful, but that you are always prepared to talk more about what the separation means to them.

❋ Do explain what will happen next (one parent moving out, for example) and how your child will still get to see each of you.

❋ Do reassure them that they are still loved by both of you: 'Even though we won't be living in the same house we will both still care for you, mind you and love you …' (This may need to be repeated regularly.)

❋ Do reassure them that the separation is not their fault and that they did nothing wrong: 'Nothing you said or did made this happen …' (This may need to be repeated regularly.)

❋ Do remember to keep acknowledging your child's good behaviour, even if they start to act out some of their upset.

❋ Do remember that telling your child is not a one-off event, but the start of a process of communicating with them about what the separation means for them.

❋ Don't criticise or blame each other in front of your children.

❋ Don't try to protect children from the hurt that the separation may bring; they need to process the difficult feelings too.

❋ Don't make a child take sides between you: they need to be able to love you both.

The trouble with hiding the truth from children

Trying to protect children from the truth of why you are separating can often do more harm than good. If adults avoid open discussion, or shut down conversations to avoid having to give information, then children infer that they shouldn't talk about what is happening. This can cause them to shut down, and leave them with many troubling feelings. While it may seem tempting to make up an explanation for the separation to satisfy their curiosity, they may overhear, or be told, the truth from another source. This can have a lasting effect on their willingness to trust their parents, who have lied to them. That trust can be hard to regain. Giving children an honest, age-appropriate explanation provides you with the opportunity to help them process their feelings, answer their questions and reassure them about their future.

How children may react

There is no single way for children to react to a family break-up. Undoubtedly the separation will cause them emotional stress so we need to remember that their first reaction may be to block their feelings. Accordingly, some children seem to react dispassionately in the early days and weeks, and may seem to be 'coping'.

Typically, though, children will experience high levels of anxiety as they accommodate the changes in their living arrangements or weekly schedules. After separation, they may have two homes, with different rules, expectations and cultures; differences between the parents are usually central to a break-up. They may take a long time to get used to the new way of living and feel displaced or up in the air.

They may also feel hurt, angry and disappointed that their parents couldn't sort out their problems. Unless they are helped to express these complicated and distressing emotions, you may find that their true feelings leak out in their behaviour or general mood. They may act angrily, aggressively or self-destructively as they, unconsciously, show you how much emotional turmoil they feel. Because children have their own personalities, temperaments and relationships with their parents, different children in the same family may show markedly different reactions to the same event.

The key is to keep trying to respond to the emotional world of your child or teenager, rather than simply reacting to their behaviour. The more they can talk openly and comprehensively about what the separation means for them, the better able they will be to accommodate the changed family circumstances successfully.

A case in point ...

The Ryan family broke up a year before they came to see me. The mum, Christine, and the dad, Terry, had finally decided to separate after years of conflict and bitter disagreement. Christine blamed Terry for working long hours and being emotionally and physically unavailable to her and their four children. Terry blamed Christine for being over-controlling and unrealistic in her expectations of him and the children.

Communication was poor between the couple, although they came to see me together. Their shared concern was for their eldest daughter, thirteen-year-old Molly, who had become disrespectful and aggressive towards Christine, to the point at which she felt unable to manage her. Christine also felt unsupported, indeed at times undermined, by Terry who was very critical of how she tried to deal with the conflicts as they arose.

Quickly I established that Terry blamed Christine for the separation, still believing that it was unnecessary. He felt she was too rigid and uncompromising and that this had also affected her relationship with the children. He was explicit in telling me that he could see why Molly hated her mum, saying that Christine was too punitive and harsh with her.

Before I spoke with Molly, I was concerned about the contrary, critical and undermining messages she was receiving from each parent about the other. I could only imagine that she was terribly confused and upset by what had happened and that her relationship with her mum was being poisoned by her dad telling her that the break-up was all her mum's fault.

I met Molly and became an emotional support for her in the midst of the ongoing conflict between her parents. She was very angry with her mum, and showed it, because she felt her mum was unyielding and never tried to understand her or see things from her perspective. She also felt angry with her dad for, as she saw it, giving up on her and her three siblings. She couldn't express this to him, though, because she was afraid that he might not want to see her.

While emotionally supporting Molly was important, it was equally important that her parents changed their behaviour. I sent Christine and Terry to counselling, independently so that each of them could begin to process the separation. At the same time, I met with them occasionally to discuss how they could still give joint-parenting messages to their children, especially Molly.

They both had to change. I got Terry to stop sympathising with Molly because, for better or worse, her mother still had the majority of time with her and needed to be authoritative. It didn't benefit Terry either to have a disrespectful daughter. I worked with Christine on empathising more with Molly and reacting to her behaviour less rigidly and punitively. As I surmised, when Molly felt better understood by her parents she had less reason to act out and her aggression disappeared.

Perhaps the most significant thing for Molly was that her parents showed, in coming to see me, that they were equally committed to her and her wellbeing. Even though she still got frustrated with her mum and still missed her dad terribly, she knew they both cared about her. She came to appreciate that they now had her best interests at heart. In the early days and months of their separation, it had been so obvious to her that each parent had been caught up in their own interpretation of the split, and she had felt lost and unnoticed.

Thankfully, Christine and Terry realised they had to put aside their disagreements and bitterness to be able to support their children. I don't think their own hurt was lessened much by the work we did, but at least they found enough common ground to allow decent and effective communication to emerge. Their own healing would come in time through their counselling, but Molly was no longer bearing the brunt of their distress and her voice was being heard.

Ensuring children don't get caught in the middle

Children may feel compromised when their parents separate. If there are high levels of animosity between the parents, children may feel they are not allowed to love the other parent because it may seem duplicitous to the parent whom they are with. For example, if a dad speaks negatively of a mum when his son is with him, it prevents the son being open about any positive feelings he has for his mother. If the child disagrees with the dad, he runs the risk of angering him, but if he agrees with his negativity, he may feel he is betraying his mother. This is a no-win situation for a child who loves both parents.

When parents are not communicating directly, as is often the case after separation, they can implicitly or explicitly use their child as a go-between. This, too, puts the child in an invidious position. As the messenger, the child may take the flak if the message is unappreciated, not accepted or misunderstood. They may be accused of taking sides as they get involved in rows and arguments that are played out through them.

Children may be appointed de facto detectives, expected to pass on information about what the other parent is up to, how they are coping, whom they are seeing, how they are spending time or money and any number of other bits of information that seem important to a parent. Children, invariably, want to be loyal to both, and to feel they are spying may make them very uncomfortable. Parents may not realise that even innocent questions can lead children to feel they are betraying a confidence or passing on information that could later be used as 'evidence' in a new conflict.

The need to mind yourself as a parent

It is possible for families to continue to thrive after separation, but only if the parents sort out their own feelings and avoid passing on their insecurity, frustration and hurt to their children. It is natural that parents will be upset and in turmoil after a break-up, but it is all too easy for their children, especially teenagers, to become their emotional support. This disrupts the natural order of things and can be a lot of pressure for a child or teenager to bear.

I advocate children taking on appropriate amounts of responsibility as they grow, but too much responsibility may be detrimental to their development. In family separation, the eldest child may often be expected to take on additional caring responsibility for younger siblings, as well as additional chores, contributing financially to the home or even to take pressure off a parent so that they don't have a 'nervous breakdown'. We need to remember that we are responsible for our children, not the other way round.

Even though parents have separated, the conflict between them may remain, so some children will continue in their role of peacekeeper. They may try, at all costs, either to stop their parents fighting or to pretend that everything is okay, even if it isn't. Neither position is emotionally sustainable for a child or teenager. They need to be able to live their own lives, not be constantly worried about everyone else's.

For parents to help children to thrive, they must deal with their own issues. The separation may have been incredibly painful, but the children need to be able to experience their own feelings, rather than be influenced by either parent. As in so many other parenting situations, the better we can mind ourselves, the better able we will be to mind our children. To support them emotionally so that they thrive again, we may need our own emotional support from outside the family.

Making it work when two families blend together

A 'blended family' is the most usual way to describe the one that forms when two adults come together with their respective children from previous relationships. It is a very common, and natural, outcome of separation, given that parents don't stop being sexual or attracted to new partners. However, in the same way that children may have felt the separation was foisted on them, setting up home with a new family is a change they don't necessarily expect or want.

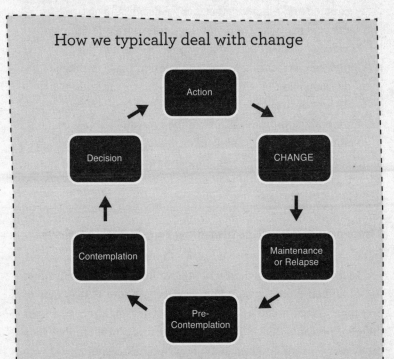

How we typically deal with change

Making change to any area of our lives is a process that follows a similar pattern for everyone.

We start in a stage of *pre-contemplation*, before we even realise that change might be necessary. Then because of life circumstances or information, we come to realise or accept that it might be on the way and we can begin to think (*contemplation*) about what it may be like. If there are enough good reasons in favour, we then make a *decision* to change. At that point we can take *action* to bring about the change. When we have made the change, we must either maintain it (in which case we exit the cycle) or we *relapse* and return to pre-contemplation.

A key aspect of any change being successfully adopted and maintained is that we decide and accept that it is necessary. Whenever we are presented with a change as a *fait accompli*, without having had the time or opportunity to contemplate and make our own decision about it, we can be resistant and even try to disrupt or derail the change that is being imposed on us. For change to occur smoothly, everyone affected by it needs a chance to think about what issues need to be resolved to achieve the change and be part of finding the necessary solutions or actions.

The opportunity that blending two families brings

It is a complex challenge to merge two families. At a practical level, you have to think about where you will live and how to accommodate the expanded family group. Should it be a house that is new to everyone? What about the interaction of the children and their different personalities? Will living together as a new family group mean some or all children moving school? Are your new living arrangements going to cause additional conflict with a previous partner? Are you ready for the commitment involved that justifies all the probable disruption?

Most importantly, given what we know about the change process, has everyone who will be affected by the merging of two families had an opportunity to talk about and be involved in the decision to make this momentous change? If not, then the complexity and impact of the change is likely to be resisted – and that resistance might be shown in a deliberate attempt by your children to scupper and disrupt the new living arrangements.

A case in point ...

William and Aoife were married with a three-year-old daughter, Grainne. William also had a son, Dominic, aged seven, from a previous relationship. Dominic lived with them every second weekend and during school holidays. William and his son had always had a very close relationship, but Aoife felt that she had never managed to 'click' with the boy. She felt he was very reserved in her company.

Aoife described how she had tried in the past to be nice to him, help him with his homework or offered to play with him, but he seemed to give nothing in return. She admitted that, consequently, she had become aloof and kept her distance because he seemed interested only in being with his father.

Dominic's withdrawal seemed to be accentuated with their daughter. He ignored her completely and didn't interact with her at all. Grainne was usually excited to see him, but this had diminished in recent months because of the constant rebuffs she received from him. Aoife described that William was very patient with his son and tried to encourage him, but did not punish him for his rudeness to her or Grainne. Aoife and William fought often about this issue since Aoife felt that Dominic should be made to interact politely with her and Grainne. The weekends when Dominic stayed over were very tense.

As we discussed the situation, it became clear to me that Aoife could not see things from Dominic's perspective so I tried to explain what his world view might be. I explained that his time with his dad was limited and, no doubt, very valuable to him. I could imagine that sharing his dad's time with Aoife could be hard. I guessed that he might resent Aoife and might blame her for taking some of his dad's precious time away. I felt that he was likely to be quite angry with her and seemed to be expressing in withdrawal and disengagement rather than open hostility and fighting.

Grainne represented a further distraction for his dad, diluting the time and attention he might receive from him. He might also *have been jealous that his sister got to live full time with his dad, but his time was comparatively limited. I could imagine that he might have felt cross with his sister about that too, further deepening his rejection of Aoife and Grainne.*

I also explained that Aoife, in many ways, mirrored Dominic's behaviour. She had grown aloof and disengaged from him, probably because she felt hurt by his snubs and rejections of her attempts to be nice to him. It seemed to me that Aoife too was being very passive-aggressive in expressing her annoyance with Dominic. Indeed, the rows between Aoife and William might well have been a displacement of Aoife's true anger towards Dominic.

Improving the family dynamic hinged on Aoife's ability to understand and deal with her own feelings of hurt at Dominic's rejection. This allowed her to get a better handle on her frustration and meant that she and William could begin to talk properly about what Dominic meant to each of them. Unsurprisingly, when they opened up, Aoife admitted she was sometimes jealous of the special bond that Dominic had with his father.

Once Aoife was more attuned to her own feelings, she was able to open up to Dominic's perspective and realised that he, too, probably had a lot of unexpressed anger and hurt. Dominic's mum refused to give permission for Dominic to come to the meetings the family had with me, so I worked closely with William and Aoife about how they could emotionally support Dominic, primarily with empathy. It was important that William, especially, actively supported Dominic to express his feelings. Like many children who don't get to live full time with a parent they love, Dominic was always nervous of being in any way negative towards, or with, his dad.

However, once William gave tacit permission, by opening the emotional conversations, it created a safer place for Dominic to be negative, without the fear that his dad would be cross with him. In fact, when William and Aoife were able to empathise with the feelings they thought he might have, it was like a dam bursting. Years of hurt poured out, about missing his dad, hating the fact that he never had time alone with him and stress about his relationship with his mum.

This was the watershed for the family and from that point they were able to heal. They had a blueprint for effective communication, and while some of the irritations persisted, they were not felt to the same degree and, most importantly, could be aired safely so that they could get on better with each other.

Common concerns for children when families merge

Children can have many and varied emotional reactions to their parents entering new relationships and making new living arrangements after a separation. If the parents have emotionally supported their child through the separation, then it is quite likely that they will also be able to help them express their feelings about blending with another family. When they can make an educated guess about the probable source of their child's feelings, it can help the child to process and deal with those feelings.

So, if you are about to merge, or have merged, your family with a new partner and their children, then one or more of the following may be an issue worth exploring with your child to understand his or her feelings:

* The separation may be seen as the fault of your new partner, who lured you away from your child's other parent, destroying your original family.
* Your new relationship, and the commitment inherent in moving in together, may underline, indeed seal, the ending of the old relationship, which may mean an end to the possible fantasy your child had of his or her parents reuniting.
* Because your child knows that you love your new partner, they may feel less loved or attended to.
* Because you now live with your new partner, your children may resent that they cannot have you all to themselves.

❊ Just because you and your partner love each other, there is no reason why your children and your partner's children should like each other – and may resent any obligation to be nice or accepting.

❊ Your child may be jealous if your partner's children live with you full time and they can't.

❊ Your child may feel that, since you have chosen to live with a new partner and their children, they no longer 'fit' in your family; they may feel displaced.

❊ Sharing you and sharing the physical space of the new home may take a lot of adjustment and may raise a lot of ire.

❊ A new partner, with or without children, can mean a new approach to parenting, which may be experienced by, and/or resented by, your child as new rules and new attitudes towards old behaviour.

Many of the potential concerns that children may harbour are either negative or may engender negative feelings. This can place them in an awkward position if they feel you will not accept their negativity. There may be no space for your child to seem negative about the new arrangements because they may fear that any criticism may lead you to love them less, or even not want to see them.

By bringing up these potential issues with your child, you show them that there is a forum within which they are allowed to be negative and that you are willing to talk about the bad stuff. Blending a family is, essentially, a process of change, so you will find that if you give your child permission and the opportunity to voice their concerns about the new family life, they will accommodate more quickly to the new arrangements.

There is always the potential for merging families to bring a lot of positive energy and vitality into children's lives. Children from different relationships can get on and can provide really positive influences and support to each other. Generally, though, they need support and time to arrive at this kind of outcome.

Dealing with death and the trauma of loss

Death is a difficult topic for any family to deal with because nothing is known about what happens to the essence of ourselves when we die. Do we have a soul or a spirit that continues some existence in a new realm? What happens after death remains a truly existential discussion, if it ever comes up for discussion at all. Children often ask questions we can't answer, and frequently we try to cover our ignorance or distract them with some other topic. Perhaps we feel their questioning is morbid or we are uncomfortable talking about death.

So, when death affects a family it is, invariably, a new thing, and many children need first to understand the concept, never mind the emotional impact of the loss it entails. How well they understand the concept is often age-related. Generally, children under the age of about five may understand that people are sad, but have no understanding of the finality of death and will see it merely as a temporary loss. Once they reach school age, and up to their pre-teens, they understand that death is permanent, but may hold on to quite concrete, generalised understanding – 'All cancer kills'; 'If I don't smoke, I won't die'; 'If my dad is "up there", then he can see me'. Usually, it is only when children reach their teens that they can understand the more abstract, existential aspects of death; they may want to debate them as part of their grieving process.

Telling a child about the death of a loved one

However you approach it, having to tell your child about the death, or imminent death, of a family member is an awful experience. It is most comforting for children to hear bad news from their parents or, at the very least, from another adult to whom they feel emotionally close. This enables them to respond naturally to the news, without feeling they have to put on a front, appear to cope, or try to protect the feelings of the person telling them.

The death of a pet: a sad but valuable lesson

Sometimes children's first experience of death is when a pet dies. Even in this situation, we can see many of the common grief reactions of sadness (often accompanied by many tears), yearning ('I wish I could stroke her fur one more time'), disbelief ('She was hardly more than a puppy, surely that's too young to die'), anger ('I hate all the drivers on the road. One of them killed her and didn't even stop!'), guilt ('I should never have let her off the lead. It's my fault she ran onto the road'), despair ('We'll never have a dog like her again') and finally, over time, reorganisation and accommodation to life without the deceased ('I heard an ad for a dog shelter that's looking for homes for their dogs – it won't be the same, but at

It is worth remembering that you will have your own powerful feelings – if the person was close to your child, they were, or are, bound to be close to you too. Some parents may not want to tell their child about something tragic, such as the death of the other parent, because they are worried that their own feelings will overwhelm the child.

In fact, our feelings won't overwhelm them as long as we don't expect them to solve our problems or make us feel better. It is important, in such situations, that children see we have other caring and supportive adults around us who will mind us, if we need to be minded. As long as children see that our emotional needs can be taken care of by another adult, it takes away any responsibility they may feel for having to look after us in the crisis.

We may be worried that our children could become insecure, following a particular bereavement, or may not cope with the enormity of the loss. This rarely happens; as long as we continue to provide the security they need, they can and will cope with our support. If you are so distraught that you aren't coping yourself, it will be reassuring for children to know that there are competent least we'd be helping some other poor dog').

Even though this is a sad time, it can be a valuable and positive lesson. If you know the pet will die (because they have to be put down) then give your child a chance to say goodbye. Then go through some of the rituals of death with your child, like saying prayers for the pet (if appropriate for your family) and burying it. This is a chance to talk about death with your child, what it means and what you believe about it. Your whole family is likely to be grieving together and this is a good thing. Talk about your dead pet often and with love. Keep a photo of the pet on the fridge, or even make a small photo album in memory. These small steps will give your child a strong foundation that will help them when faced with the death of a person they love.

adults available who seem to be coping okay and will ensure that the children's needs will be met. Do bring in extended family or close family friends, who can be there for your children if you, emotionally, can't be at that moment.

By telling children, and regularly making space to talk about what has happened, we let them know that death is not a taboo subject and is not so awful that it cannot, or should not, be talked about. This gives them the freedom to ask more questions or to bring the subject up again as part of their grieving process.

It helps to tell children as much as possible about what has happened (or what is likely to happen) so that they can begin to adjust to the changes that will inevitably occur. The sooner you can tell children about definite losses, like death or incurable illness, the better.

Children will be very sensitive to your emotions and if you delay telling them (believing that you are protecting them), they may sense that something is wrong . If you don't tell them what it is, they may become unnecessarily distressed about some imagined trauma. Once they know, their distress will be appropriately focused and they can begin to grieve fully.

If you delay telling your child about some major crisis that affects your family, they may find out by default, from an overheard conversation or someone outside the family, which may leave them resentful that they weren't told and terrified that there is more they don't know.

Involving children in the rituals of death

I believe it is better for children to be as fully involved as possible in whatever rituals – such as wakes, removals, funerals, burials or cremations – their family is following. It may be tempting to exclude youngsters, on the basis that they will be upset or because they won't know what's going on, but it has been found repeatedly that missing out on the rituals of death complicates the grieving process for children. Even if you feel you can't be emotionally present enough to support your children during the funeral, assign that role to another family member so that your child can be present. Unfortunately children and adults have to experience intense upset and sadness as part of their ultimate healing.

A case in point ...

Jamie was ten and his father had died of cancer the year before he came to see me. During the first session, Gwen, his mother, was extremely tearful in recounting her husband's illness, his apparent remission from the cancer and then the devastating news that the cancer had returned. He died within two weeks of the secondary diagnosis. While she was speaking, I noticed that Jamie either didn't look at her, or shot her angry, disapproving glances.

His difficulties were two-fold. He had become entirely disrespectful to his mother, cursing at her, calling her names and hitting her, but alternating this with genuine caring and affection. This confused and distressed Gwen terribly as she never knew whether she would meet the 'devil or the sweetheart'. At the same time, Jamie was in significant trouble in school where he and his teacher regularly ended up in shouting matches before Jamie was dispatched to the principal's office for his 'insolence'.

I met with Jamie's teacher and the school principal at his mother's request and discovered that they were finding him almost unmanageable. They acknowledged his bereavement and felt they had been accommodating in the months following his father's death, and very lenient with him whenever he erupted in the class. Now they felt that his current behaviour was more likely to relate to ODD (Oppositional Defiant Disorder). I completely disagreed.

Before his father's death Jamie had been lively in class but never disobedient. He had no history of ODD. His really challenging behaviour had only started during his father's illness and continued after his death. I explained the likely grieving process and the typical timescales (it can take a child a number of years to move through their grief at the loss of a parent) that Jamie might be experiencing. I strongly believed that his behaviour in school was a reaction to his father's death and needed to be responded to as such.

It was significant, too, that his teacher was a man. It was quite likely that Jamie struggled with a male authority figure because this man might trigger further his sense of loss. His father had played a very authoritative role at home and Jamie might have felt echoes of his father every time his teacher challenged his behaviour. The anger that Jamie probably felt about his father's death became directed at his teacher instead.

Armed with their new understanding, his teacher and the principal agreed to try a range of interventions to help Jamie. These included:

❋ *Focusing intensely on opportunities to 'catch him being good'*

❋ *Trying to be specific in identifying any positive behaviour that supported the class or his own learning*

❋ *Remaining firm, but understanding, with him if his behaviour was unacceptable or potentially dangerous for himself or others*

❋ *Trying to empathise with his distress and anger, knowing they were still fuelled by grief, with the aim of reducing the intensity of any outbursts*

❋ *Offering him opportunities to be out of the class for short periods with the resource teacher*

❋ *Offering him opportunities to take on responsibility within the class*

❋ *Involving Jamie in an after-school chess club, run by his teacher, so that they could have fun together outside the rules and structures of the class and build a more positive relationship.*

At the same time, I continued to see Jamie individually. We spent many sessions talking about his dad and the real tragedy of his death. Jamie carried a strong resentment because he hadn't been told initially about the illness. When his dad had started losing his hair during chemotherapy, Jamie had guessed that something was wrong and asked his mother, who eventually told him about the cancer. Jamie believed strongly that if he had known from the start, he wouldn't have been so cheeky to his dad and wouldn't have caused him the stress that he believed had caused the return of the cancer. It took many sessions before Jamie was able to accept that his dad's death was not his fault.

Jamie felt the loss of his dad intensely. He had been very close to him. Jamie was always on the go and his dad had always tried to keep him busy. He had been a farmer and Jamie had spent many hours with him on the land. 'He was my best friend,' was *how Jamie described him. In contrast, he had little time for his mother who, he felt, had never understood him. During one session, Jamie angrily pronounced that he wished his mother had died, not his father, because he wouldn't miss her so much. Although it may seem shocking, it made sense and it was an issue that, once voiced, we could work on to help strengthen his relationship with her without the resentment.*

Jamie did work through the anger he felt about the injustice of his dad's death and his sense that he had been cheated of his relationship with such a profoundly central figure in his life. He settled again in school, helped by renewed understanding and patience from his teacher. His relationship with his mum stayed tricky for a long while, in part because his mum was also grieving and emotionally unavailable to him at times. But she, too, began healing, with her own therapeutic support and the benefit of time. They still fought but it seemed fairer, and Jamie was less dismissive of and disrespectful to her. When I last saw Jamie, he had just become a teenager and most of their rows seemed like normal family life to me.

Having time to say goodbye

When children and adults have an opportunity to say goodbye to a person who is dying, it can be a very healing experience. It can't always happen because some deaths are sudden and unexpected. When children do get to say goodbye, however, it gives them a chance to review and acknowledge the good or positive things that will be lost and express their feelings about it with the person. Painful though it may feel at the time, the dying person can give their blessing and overt permission for the child to move on (in time) and have a full, satisfying and successful life without them. This kind of considered and emotionally real goodbye can relieve a lot of future guilt and obligation and tends to leave a lot less unfinished business that might otherwise complicate the grief that will follow.

Understanding the grieving process

In many ways, there is no such thing as a typical grief experience because every person is different and will go through the grieving process in a different way. There are, however, several stages or phases of grief that everyone will experience. Each stage is typified by a particular feeling. What varies is the order in which the stages and feelings occur and the length of time spent working through each feeling.

Common feelings during grieving

* Shock, disbelief and denial
* Yearning and pining
* Sadness
* Anger
* Worry and anxiety
* Guilt
* Shame
* Hopelessness and despair
* Accommodation: reorganising and engaging with life in a new way.

Children may have a mixture of these feelings, although usually one feeling predominates at any time. They can shift between the feelings, and as one subsides another may quickly take its place. Grieving is a slow process; moving through all these stages and recovering from the loss may take children several years, sometimes longer. The process may be intermittent, too, with breaks of seeming normality or coping. During this time, children need to know that their feelings are the normal feelings of grief and to be reassured that things will get easier, even if they don't believe you.

Many parents, coping with their own grief, cannot tolerate these feelings being expressed by their children, and may try to suppress them, particularly if they lead to behaviour that seems destructive or harmful. This makes the process harder for children and may mean they need someone outside the family to help them to express their true feelings and work through them.

Similarly, some children will see the deep distress of their parent(s) and feel that they cannot add to that distress with their own feelings. They may try to hide or block them, reluctant or unwilling to express them because they fear it will make a bad situation worse – this only destabilises an already struggling parent. Again, it is crucial that another care-giving adult is available for emotional and even practical support in these circumstances.

The ideas given at the start of this chapter (see page 240) about helping children to understand and express their feelings will be helpful during their grieving. Authentic empathy and respect from caring adults supports them in their progression through the different feelings they are likely to encounter. We need to be patient and allow them to feel their emotions as they surface. We may wish to rush them through, get them to stop being angry, for example, but actually we need to give them time and understanding.

Coping with serious illness

Illness is a threat to thriving within a family. Even a child with a cold, who is not at school or with their carer, creates extra pressure for parents who may have to take time off work, never mind worrying about the illness. When a serious illness affects anyone in a family the stresses within the family are magnified considerably.

Unless we have grown up in a family with a sick parent or sibling, it is quite likely that the experience of dealing with a serious illness is new. Even our understanding of the disease may be minimal and we need to equip ourselves with as much information as possible. Understanding a diagnosis, or a prognosis for the likely development of the illness, can be upsetting, and difficult to absorb.

If a husband, wife or partner has become ill, we will probably have extra domestic and financial responsibility. Depending on how the roles were shared before the illness, this may be extremely challenging. If a child is sick, parents are likely to take it in turns to be focused on the care or companionship of the child, leaving the other parent to run the rest of the family.

The varying responses

Everyone in the family will have some kind of emotional response to the illness. For example, while one parent undergoes tests and treatments, such as surgery or therapy, and tries to cope with symptoms, such as pain, breathlessness or loss of a part of their body or its function, the other parent may be feeling shocked, angry, helpless, in disbelief and doubting their ability to deal with so many changes.

No matter who in the family is sick – parent or child – there may be fear and worry about the future. It is easy for parents and children to feel out of control and distressed with many changes and little certainty. Many families may feel disorganised and have a hard time adjusting to new routines or restrictions imposed by the illness. Depending on the nature of the illness and its prognosis, family members may be sad, even depressed and hopeless, about how their lives have been altered.

As with other traumas that affect families, the key is to talk early and often about what the illness means to each family member and what kinds of feelings children and parents are experiencing. Subjugating feelings to get through the days and complete the tasks of keeping a family going is common. Support from extended family or friends can give parents the time and opportunity to fall apart emotionally, if that is what they need to do for short periods, safe in the knowledge that other adults can take on the caring role.

Coping mechanisms

* Recognise your own feelings and reactions to the illness within the family. These changes in your mood can have an impact on how you react to non-illness-related issues too.
* Recognise that the sick person is also experiencing huge emotional and psychological stress, as well as the physical toll of the illness. This may affect how they behave towards the rest of the family.
* Have regular family meetings that incorporate opportunities for everyone to offload the stress, worries, fears and frustrations that the illness is provoking.
* Gather as much information as you can about the illness, the treatment (if any), and its physical and psychological impact.
* Try to remain hopeful, without closing down opportunities to talk about 'what if …' scenarios.
* Work to maintain friendships, and relationships with extended family, who are supportive both emotionally and practically.
* Be realistic in planning for your own needs and other responsibilities. Frequently reassess your 'care load' and ask for the help you need without feeling guilty. Minding yourself and having time off is important. You don't have to be all things to all people. Doing too much will lead to stress and burn-out.
* Talk to your employer if the illness is having an impact on your attendance or performance at work. The more you can explain and contextualise your behaviour, the more understanding and helpful an employer can be.
* Seek new ways to interact with the ill person if activities shared previously are no longer possible because of the progressive physical or psychological nature of the illness.
* Remember that other family members have needs, as well as the person who is ill. While you may not be able to meet them all, you may be able to find ways for others to help.

A case in point ...

Giles and Sandra were parents to a three-year-old daughter, Caoimhe, and a one-year-old son, Feidhlim. Feidhlim was born with cystic fibrosis (CF) and had spent a lot of his first year in hospital. Sandra had left work to care for him. She wanted to help him to cope with the extra challenges he would have to face because of his illness and the routines of medication and physiotherapy each day. She worried his life would not be normal, yet she didn't want to spoil him.

One of the most important things that Giles and Sandra needed to do was spend time as a couple, and as individuals, thinking and talking about what Feidhlim's illness meant for each of them. They needed to come to terms with the fact of his shorter life expectancy and the realisation that his life probably wouldn't be the same as others'. Sandra, for example, acknowledged that he was different and that he would need a treatment regime, but accepting that he was different meant acknowledging the disappointment, grief or loss she may have felt about whatever expectations of normality she had anticipated before his birth.

Giles had quite a different take on the CF and its impact as he had grown up with a brother who had died from CF, aged just twenty-two. He was fully aware of the physiotherapy and other treatments that were involved because he had watched Struan struggle. He had watched his mother devote herself to him. Even at our first meeting, there was a hint of resentment in his tone as he described his mum's care for his brother. Indeed, Giles was equally worried about Caoimhe and what impact Feidhlim's condition would have on her, as he believed that he had suffered because of his own brother's CF.

As part of our discussions, we looked at the likelihood of Feidhlim being able to participate as fully as other children in many activities. I encouraged them to focus, with him, as he got older, on the things he would be able to do, rather than things he would not, to support him in having a more positive outlook on life and on what was achievable, even with CF.

We talked about how, like every child, they would need to set limits for Feidhlim as he got a bit older. They still needed to determine the boundaries for his behaviour and make sure he learned the rules of the house. It might have been tempting to try to compensate for some of the complexity or distress he might experience by being lenient or laissez-faire with him, but they both realised this wouldn't help him in the long term.

Giles's awareness of the impact on siblings meant he advocated balancing out their parental time and attention between both children. Initially, this was harder for Sandra because she was so caught up with the medical issues that had kept Feidhlim in and out of the hospital for his first year. But, as she got to talk to other parents of children with CF, she realised he wasn't in imminent danger of 'breaking'. This gave her the time and space to consider Caoimhe more.

Since Sandra was at home so much, she made sure she gave Caoimhe the opportunity to be with her one-to-one. Playing with Caoimhe not only gave Sandra the chance to give her the attention she needed, but insights into how her daughter was feeling: Caoimhe liked to play some very rough and angry games!

The only other advice I gave them was to make sure to keep talking to each other. It might have been easy for Giles and Sandra to fall into roles and habits, and to assume that each knew how the other felt about all that was going on. Ongoing anxieties, stresses and challenges were quite likely for their family, so the more that Giles and Sandra could mind themselves and each other, the better able they would be to help their children thrive.

The impact on siblings

In my experience, siblings often face significant challenges and have a range of complex feelings about the ill child. Not all of the feelings are positive. Common negative feelings that siblings may have include:

❋ **Fear/worry** – that their brother or sister might die or be in real pain and discomfort

❋ **Jealousy** – that their sibling receives all of the attention in the house from parents and visitors

❋ **Anger** – that their needs don't seem to be as important

❋ **Resentment** – that they may have extra responsibility, or may have to care for their brother or sister, or that they may not be able to do certain things because their sibling's needs take priority

❋ **Embarrassment** – at how their sibling looks or acts

❋ **The weight of additional expectations** – perhaps they are expected to do, or be, what their sibling cannot do or be

❋ **Guilt** – for having negative feelings (which may not be acceptable to parents); they may also feel guilty for not being sick and not having the challenges that their sibling has.

Parents' inability to accept any negativity about the ill child can be a real block to their other children's healthy development and functioning. Having to deny such understandably negative feelings will lead a child or teenager to get stuck with those feelings and they are quite likely to act out the emotional hurt in challenging or self-destructive behaviour.

When parents can allow, and indeed encourage, the expression of all of the feelings, positive and negative, that a child has about a sick or disabled sibling, he or she has space to thrive. In fact, such siblings typically grow up with many positive attributes that can be a direct result of their experience with an ill sibling. Through caring or standing up for their brother or sister they may grow to be:

❋ More patient

❋ More tolerant and understanding of difference

❋ More responsible or dependable

❋ More compassionate and empathetic

❋ Kinder and more thoughtful.

But, as in many family situations, sometimes the negative feelings have to be expressed before the positive ones can find their expression.

Allowing emigration to be an opportunity for a thriving family

There are many reasons why families choose to uproot and move to a new country. Sometimes the choice is unavoidable and the result of economic necessity; sometimes it is freely made for a perceived better lifestyle or other quality-of-life reasons. Whatever a family's motivation, the move involves many changes for everyone involved.

In that context, distress and worry are natural emotions. Just as small children can be destabilised by changes to their routine, the unpredictability that comes with emigration may lead any, or all, family members to feel insecure and fearful of the unknown elements of their future lives. Different family members may also have different fears, or may worry about some things more intensely than others. For example, one child may be worried about making new friends and another about missing old ones.

Emigration within the EU may not be complex, in that EU citizens do not require visas to live or work elsewhere in the EU. However, language may be a much more significant challenge for everyone. Emigration to the US, Canada, Australia and similar countries has the benefit of sharing a language but may have a long-drawn-out and complicated visa application process. No matter which country a family considers moving to, there will be significant cultural differences to which each person must adapt.

Coping with the response

In anticipation of the widespread changes in a family's circumstances, resistance to moving is common. Typically parents instigate the emigration process; they have realised that change is necessary

Practical tips to reduce children's and teenagers' resistance and ease their transition

* **Talk to them early.** Include them in the discussion as early as is practical so you can explain your rationale for moving and why you think it will be better for your family.
* **Be honest about what the move entails.** Be realistic with them about missing friends and family, about having to change school, about learning a new language or adapting to a new culture.
* **Encourage them to express their feelings.** Try to help them describe the good and bad feelings they may have about the move. Listen empathetically, without rushing to try to fix any perceived problems they may predict. This may not be a single conversation but one of many over the months of preparation for moving.
* **Balance their worries.** The chances are that children and teenagers will see the problems with emigrating sooner than they will spot the possibilities it offers. As long as you allow them to express the negative feelings, it is okay to balance this with reassurances about the exciting opportunities for them and for the family as a whole.

and come to the decision that emigration is the best option, or action, to achieve it. As long as they are of one mind, and keep talking about the process with each other, they should remain equally committed to the move.

By the time they discuss their decision with their children, they have usually tossed the idea back and forth many times and have come to terms with it. Children, however, may feel the move has

- ❈ **Provide lots of information about the country you are migrating to.** Use DVDs, brochures and the Internet to find out about what is on offer, including things to see and do, to spark their interest and enthusiasm for the potential benefits.

- ❈ **Involve them in the planning.** Depending on the children's ages, let them look through rental property details, school brochures or information about clubs and societies they may join. This enables them to feel greater control and ownership of what will happen and may reduce their worries.

- ❈ **Take advantage of familiarity.** With younger children you can bring favoured toys, small items of furniture or trinkets that keep some continuity with the home they know. For older children and teenagers you can also maintain continuity with their sports or pastimes in the new country.

- ❈ **Consider developing pen-pals in the country to which you are moving.** Having email or written contact with children or teenagers of their age can mean a ready-made friend when they arrive.

- ❈ **Reassure them about maintaining contact with friends and family.** Remind them of the many options for keeping in touch with those people that they may miss (phone calls, Skype, emails, social networking, letters and text messages).

been foisted upon them. They may not have been expecting the announcement, or feel that emigrating is the best answer to their current family circumstances. They will be several steps back in the process and may not even accept that any change, never mind such radical change, is necessary.

If this is so, they may be very resistant to emigrating; they may be worried about what they will lose by leaving and/or what life will be like in the new country. They may also resist because they feel they were not consulted and don't agree with the decision.

Openness, honesty, time and regular discussions about all aspects of the planned move will help to reduce, and even dissipate, their resistance. As long as children feel they are listened to and understood, their initial resistance may shift to excitement about the opportunities ahead.

A case in point ...

Jane fell in love with an Australian, Rob, who had been living in Ireland for a year. Unexpectedly they had a daughter, who had turned five by the time Jane came to see me. She and Rob had never married and their relationship was somewhat on and off. Becky, their daughter, proved to be the glue that usually reunited them if their rows ever split them up. However, Rob was putting pressure on Jane to move to Australia with him as he felt they would have more opportunities there and that they would be a family more successfully. Jane didn't doubt Rob's love for her or for Becky and couldn't really imagine Becky not growing up with her dad.

She found making the decision about possibly emigrating wearing, though, and came to me for advice. She went to and fro in her mind about what would be best for Becky. Since Rob seemed determined to go, she was afraid that Becky would lose her relationship with her dad if they didn't travel with him. She also acknowledged that she couldn't get work here and that they were under constant financial pressure, which also contributed to the fights between herself and Rob. On the other hand, Becky had just settled into school and had a really supportive network of friends and cousins. Jane, too, liked the emotional support that her extended family offered.

This was a real dilemma for her. I encouraged her to make a list of the pros and cons of moving to Australia as there were clear costs and benefits with each choice. Unfortunately for her, by the end of the exercise she still felt caught between a rock and a hard place. Practically, staying at home seemed wiser, but emotionally, she wanted her relationship with Rob to work out and for Becky to maintain her wonderfully close relationship with her dad. Ultimately her heart won out and she decided to emigrate.

Two years later, Jane was back to see me, tearfully describing how her relationship with Rob had ended and that she and Becky were back home without him. She described how she had never settled in Australia and that Rob had fallen back into his old life with his buddies, leaving her feeling more neglected. She came to resent the huge sacrifices she had made and felt at a loss to cope without her own family to lean on.

As we discussed the process, it was clear that Jane had been most persuaded to move by her desire to keep Rob as an active father in Becky's life but that, ultimately, this aspiration had not proved to be enough to sustain all the pressures of emigrating. It had been a really painful experience and now she was picking up the pieces as she and Becky came to terms with the separation from Rob and resettling back home.

The need for clarity and honesty

It's hard to sell a move to your children unless you're clear about why you're moving. For some emigrants, the move is tantamount to running away from problems; they believe that marital stress or disharmony, for example, will disappear with greater financial stability or a change of scenery. In fact, the stresses of moving may lead to the fracture of an already distressed marriage.

It can really help to do a cost-benefit analysis, comparing the positives and negatives of emigration. Write down all the positive reasons why you should move in one column, and all the negatives in another beside it. You can either see which list is the longer or you can assign each reason (positive and negative) a score or a rating to reflect its relative importance. This is an inexact but helpful indicator of where the balance lies in favour of or against moving. Emigrating must offer more benefits than costs.

It also helps to write down all of your hopes and expectations about what might be possible in the new country. This will also serve as a positive reminder of the opportunities that exist, or may exist. Having a positive frame of reference (reminding yourself why you wanted to do this!) can lift your spirits and may also enable you to remain positive and supportive for the rest of your family. This helps when the going is tough in the lead-up to the move or in the early days when everything is in a bit of a heap while you're starting to settle.

Job loss as a motivator for emigration

If life at home changes radically because either or both parents become unemployed or have poor job prospects, it can be tempting to think about opportunities that might exist abroad. However, before considering moving to a new country, it is worth spending time accommodating to your changed circumstances at home.

Becoming unemployed is a very significant loss for anybody who has experienced it. When you lose your job, you may feel that you have also lost your social status, professional identity, lifestyle, social contacts, weekly structure or routine, sense of security and self-confidence. It is easy to feel numbed, angry, upset and anxious about any or all of these factors.

Getting away to a new life in a new country may seem like a panacea, but it may also be a distraction or a way of dissociating from the real pain and distress of becoming unemployed. Emigration may be a consideration down the line, when you feel you are coming to terms with the losses of unemployment. In the early stages, however, you need to give yourself time to grieve, as with any other loss, and to get used to your new family circumstances.

Settling in

The biggest factors for your children settling in are likely to be their ease in making friends and settling into school. In both cases, it is important to be realistic about the challenges involved. They may find themselves at a loss to communicate effectively, which can dent their usual confidence – especially if language is a barrier. Do focus on tuition and help to learn the language as quickly as possible.

Finding common interests with peers really helps this transition, so enrolling your children in after-school clubs or activities they enjoy may connect with other children in a natural and enjoyable way. Activities such as football, dance and swimming can be like a common language. When children realise that they share common interests or passions, they tend to be welcoming and work hard to overcome obstacles, such as awkward communication. A smile is also understood around the world, and when children approach situations with a positive attitude and a willingness to be friendly, it tends to be reciprocated.

The curriculum in the new school may be quite different from that which they left, so do keep in close contact with your child's teacher(s) to ensure that homework remains manageable. Equally, if homework is too challenging, explain to the teachers where the difficulties lie. Most schools will be willing to find the right balance between what is achievable and what is expected.

Take advantage, too, of the things you love about your new country. Arranging trips to places of natural beauty or high-adrenalin fun (like theme or water parks) gives everyone a break from the mundane tasks of settling in and is a helpful reminder of the positive opportunities your move can offer.

The most important thing is to keep talking to each other about the challenges or difficulties you are facing. Everyone in the family might be finding different aspects of the move tough. Being open to problem-solving ideas and remaining understanding will make settling in easier for everyone. It takes time to get used to difference and for things to become familiar and predictable, but families do accommodate, successfully, to living abroad. Sometimes patience, time and a positive attitude are all you need.

07

CONTINUING TO THRIVE WHEN CHILDREN BECOME ADULTS

Entering adulthood: accommodating the move into full emotional and psychological independence

The transition to adulthood is another significant developmental step that we all make. We can sometimes forget, in our focus on the family we have created, that we are already the adult children of our parents. They have been through this transitional phase with us. How we relate to them, as adults, is affected by their behaviour and our own.

Because we are the adult children of our parents, and will, in turn, become the parents of adult children, we need to look at the experience of this stage in family life from both perspectives. The main goal that marks the transition to adulthood is to become emotionally and psychologically separate from your parents so that you can assume a responsible independence. Two interlinking processes affect this.

On the one hand, the young adult must pull themselves apart from the emotional and psychological world of their parents; on the other, the parents must push the young adult to be responsibly independent of them. There can be resistance, reluctance and blocks to the process from both the young adult and the parent.

Separating psychologically from your parents

There is, typically, a period of unease while we renegotiate the relationship between our parents and ourselves. It is not always easy for our parents, who may not recognise that they have to treat us differently.

Ideally we need to create opportunities for dialogue where we can be heard, old hurts from either side can be acknowledged and healed, and we can find new and positive ways of relating, as equal adults.

An underlying theme in this book has been how the experiences that we have as children growing up profoundly affect the kind of adults, and parents, we become. Knowing our history helps us to make sense of our present behaviour, attitudes and feelings.

Our histories may be complex, however. Our parents were human, which means they were imperfect and made mistakes. When we become adults, we can hold strong feelings, even resentment, towards our parents that will influence the kind of adult relationship we have with them. Some of the mistakes they made will have affected us negatively. Such experiences can vary hugely, from regular family stress to more chronic or complex difficulties. Perhaps you grew up in a home where a parent was an alcoholic or a gambler; perhaps they were physically or sexually abusive. Any or all of these kinds of parental failings have a huge impact on the children who grow up in that environment. Your experience with your family of origin may have meant that you didn't thrive. Indeed, you may feel that you barely survived.

Arising from such experiences, you may, in your current life, have issues with trust, guilt, shame, fear, aggression or a range of other feelings that are a direct outcome of the betrayal, abuse and terror you experienced as a child. It is hard to feel like a separate and independent adult when so much of your emotional world and your behaviour are enmeshed with your childhood experiences and your complicated relationship with your parents.

Even if situations were not traumatically abusive, we carry a legacy from how our parents treated us to the extent that we can still remain emotionally dependent on them. Not only do we need to be 'let go' by our parents, we also have to detach and separate ourselves from them to become fully independent adults in our own right. That means that we have to set boundaries on our behaviour and make decisions about our own lives. It can mean challenging our parents' continuing influence on – or their attempt to influence – our behaviour and us. It means taking full responsibility for our actions, including the consequences of the mistakes that we will inevitably make. In essence, our relationships with our parents must become adult-to-adult relationships, rather than child-to-parent relationships.

Creating healthy adult relationships with our parents

We have to move on emotionally, psychologically and physically from our role of being a child. Let's not kid ourselves that this is an easy task, or that just because we know it must be done we have the skills or motivation to do it. Accepting your adulthood and standing on your own in the world involves loss – most especially, the loss of nurture and closeness.

We also lose the irresponsibility that childhood gave us. When we made mistakes as a child or teenager, our parents were probably there to pick up the pieces and mediate the consequences. The true sign of adulthood is accepting full responsibility for our actions and ourselves. We have to be ready and willing to take on this responsibility.

With luck, your parents will be doing their part to help you to grow fully into your adulthood but, if not, you may need to reflect (as part of your own personal development or therapeutic work) and make any necessary changes alone. The following steps will help you to set boundaries and establish yourself as an adult and should help you to carve out a new and positive relationship with your parents.

'Failure to launch' and the 'boomerang generation'

'Failure to launch' is a term used to describe those adult offspring who never leave their family home, although they may be in their late twenties or early thirties. The 'boomerang generation' refers to those adults who, having left home to go to college or get work, return to the family home because of financial hardship or to save money.

Having adult children in your home, or being the adult child at home with your parents, requires a significant shift in the dynamic that existed when the children were actually children and teenagers. Young adults who continue to live at home may fall into the trap of expecting their parents to continue to meet their emotional needs (for example, including them in dinner plans or keeping the home a nurturing place in which they are minded), while also expecting their parents to grant them independence of behaviour.

This is a very difficult dynamic to balance on both parts. Adult children may seek to protect the limited responsibility of childhood yet want the privileges that come with adulthood. A parent who is expected to continue to nurture will also still expect to set rules and boundaries so that they don't feel their children are taking advantage of them. An adult child will not want to give up the luxuries of home life and may resent the

Be an adult when you are with your parents

It is so easy to walk back into your parents' house, feel like a small child again and act like one. They are unlikely to be ready to treat you differently, so you must treat them differently. Feeling and acting like an adult in the company of your parents is key to consequences of this, which are that they will still be treated as a child.

It is not emotionally or developmentally healthy for adult children to remain at home. No matter the bargaining, or the payment of rent or subsistence, the tensions between parents and adult children over core issues like responsibility will rumble on. Ultimately, neither the parent nor the adult child matures into their next developmental stage.

The key is for both the parents and the adult children to have a desire for living independently of each other. The recent economic hardships or job losses that many young adults have experienced may have prompted a grateful and understandable return to their parents' home and support. When this move home is seen as a temporary arrangement it can be functional, and no parent is going to want their son or daughter to experience unnecessary hardship.

However, when adult children are reluctant to go and are not pulling themselves, developmentally, forward, they need a push. As adults, we need to do things for ourselves, not remain dependent on our parents to fill in the gaps. If we still look to our parents to solve our problems, we are not thriving on our own resources. If we are not internally motivated to thrive on our own resources, we may need the external pressure of being 'encouraged' out of the home.

having an adult relationship with them. When you talk to them, for example, talk like an adult. It can help to pause and think about how you might respond if a friend said the same thing to you that your mother or father just said. Then respond or behave as if it was to a friend.

Share your adult life with them

Unless your parents get a sense from you about who you are in the world, how you interact and what you do, they cannot get a new perspective on you and will continue to deal with you as they did when you were younger. Unless they know about your life outside their home, they can only continue to relate to you about family issues. They need the new context of your life to have an expanded view of you. This will also allow you and them to have things to talk about that are not about family.

Make your own decisions

When we ask for advice from our parents, we may actually be asking for their approval. This is a very typical dynamic that is established in childhood because parental approval is vital to a child's sense of security. By continuously, or regularly, asking for advice in adulthood, we continue to give the message that we are not responsible. Indeed, it may reflect our insecurity about being an adult in the world and our doubts about our ability to cope.

Your parents may give unsolicited advice and you can listen respectfully (they probably have your best interests at heart) but you can still feel free to make your own decision, without guilt.

Solve your own problems

It may be tempting to ring your mother and see if she'll pick up your children because you have been delayed at work. Perhaps your parents seem like an obvious first choice for a financial bail-out if times are tight. But every time you rely on their support (which they will usually give happily), you fall back into old dependencies and old parent–child roles. If you keep relying on your parents to help you cope in the world, you will never thrive in your own right.

Set clear boundaries

Your parents may pass judgement about aspects of your life and how you are living it, but you don't have to accept it. When your parents criticise and belittle your choices, they will sap your self-esteem unless you challenge them. If you are truly adult, you can say, 'Stop,' to your parents. Sometimes we have to draw a line and acknowledge that we will not discuss certain topics because they cause too much pain.

It is important to hang on to what is meaningful to you and not to change or compromise who you are just to make your parents happy. There is nothing wrong with having different values or beliefs from them, and you can continue to respect your parents' choices as you would like them to respect yours. They may, in fact, be judging you as a way of coping with their loss of control now that you have taken your life into your own hands.

Recognising that your children are adults and thriving when they move on

Hopefully, you have successfully renegotiated your relationship with your parents and can relate to them in an adult way. If so, your next challenge is the other side of the coin: renegotiating your relationship with your child who has become an adult.

At different stages on our children's developmental paths, we may feel that the difficult stages will end and that parenting and the relationship we have with our children will become less challenging. At times when we struggle with aspects of our children's behaviour or with their moods, we may long for the 'greener grass' that is bound to lie ahead when they are older: 'Once he can talk, it'll be easier to deal with him'; 'I'll have more time when I'm not changing nappies all day'; 'She'll settle down once she gets into school'; 'It'll be great when he has different subject teachers in secondary school and isn't so negative about the one teacher'; 'As soon as she reaches eighteen, I no longer have to be responsible for her.'

What we come to realise as our children grow older is that issues do change but that, typically, as one challenge subsides another takes its place. This is because children and teenagers are always in some state of developmental progression, and will change their attitudes and behaviour as they mature and their circumstances change. When your children reach adulthood, their developmental progression continues so we have to continue to adapt to the changing landscape of our relationship with them.

In a thriving family, children will have taken on more responsibility for themselves and their behaviour as they matured. They will have had opportunities to trust and be trusted. They will have been respected and will have matured to become respectful teenagers and young adults. In a thriving family, the whole thrust of the parents' work will have been to hold their children close (physically, emotionally and psychologically) as babies and toddlers and, gradually, let them go to inhabit the physical, emotional and psychological world outside the family.

The more experience that children, teenagers and young adults have of the world, the more they can test and refine their own values to form their identities and become fully independent of us. This is what we are aiming for, yet ironically it is also what many of us continue to resist long after we could have allowed our adult children to be independent.

Coping with the sense of loss

I think there is always a degree of loss to be suffered by parents as their children move into each developmental phase. Most of us will have the mixed feelings of delight at our child going to school for the first time, but also perhaps a tinge of regret that we are no longer the only big influence on them or that they no longer need us in the same way.

Many of us resist the changes that will come as our children and teenagers become less dependent on us. We may have become comfortable in our roles as providers, nurturers, guides, and so on, and don't necessarily want to give up those roles. Sometimes our own adult identity changed when we became parents, and being a parent may now define who we are.

It is natural for parents to be slow to move on. Most parents will try to preserve the same relationship that they had with their children when they were young, even if they then go on to complain about how their children don't seem to be growing up. In truth, the parents may not be letting them grow up.

Accepting that our adult children are independent radically alters our parenting role and means that we have to create a new identity for ourselves. We don't stop being a parent, but we need to find a new way to relate to our adult child. Our relationship with our adult offspring is not the same as that with other adults because our sons and daughters will always be our sons and daughters – they are just no longer our children. The shift may leave us bereft and at a loss to know how to be with, and how to relate to, our adult child in the interim.

Empty-nest syndrome

Empty-nest syndrome is the term coined to describe the feelings of loss and sadness that parents may have when their children leave home. Many parents are not prepared for the vacuum this may create. Mothers and fathers may have based their self-worth or sense of value on their role as a care-giver and parent. When that role is not needed to the same extent, it can leave them feeling worthless and even depressed.

The time that you will have when your children finally leave is an opportunity, but being prepared is the key. In fact, more mothers than fathers prepare emotionally for their children leaving. Men tend not to see it as a particularly important transition and may be surprised by the loss they feel. Men, in fact, are more likely to prepare for retirement than they are to prepare for life without their children.

Preparation minimises the impact of children leaving although you have to experience it before you can fully understand how it will affect you. Some of the following suggestions may help you prepare.

* **Make a list of how you can spend your free (and quiet!) time.** We all have moments in the hurly-burly of family life when we long for a quiet moment to be able to do something nurturing for ourselves. This may be the time to start writing that novel, reading a book by an author you admire, knitting the jumper you have promised yourself for years, organising all the photos on the computer and printing the best ones, or any number of other activities.

* **Travel.** Your adult child or children are broadening their horizons by moving out and this creates a real opportunity for you to do the same. Get out the brochures or go online. Read some travel literature to inspire yourself.

* **Focus on your friendships.** Maintaining close friendships takes time and energy and many friends may have been on your emotional back-burner while you were busy with your children. You also have time to develop new friendships, perhaps to be found in evening classes, sports clubs and drama groups.

* **Find something meaningful and valuable to do.** To keep your self-esteem high, it's important to feel valued and capable. In many ways you need to replace the fulfilment you may have got from being a hands-on parent. Your skills and talents will be welcomed in any number of voluntary groups. Look at charities you have supported financially and see if they would have a use for your time instead. Look to your church or local community to see what might appeal to you.

Allowing grandparents to be a thriving part of your family

When you became a parent, you elevated your own parents to a new position – that of grandparent. This is another central feature of most people's adult relationships with their parents. The most important thing to remember about grandparenting is that grandparents have their own unique relationship with your children. They are not an extension of you.

Depending on your relationship with your parents, you may or may not welcome their involvement, as a grandparent, in the life of your family. Even if you have had your own difficult times with them, you may discover that they have changed and that they take on a very different role with your children than they ever did with you. I think it really benefits children to have a strong connection to their extended family. Grandparents may be very important people in their lives.

The importance of grandparents

There has been a lot of research into the important roles that older adults in general, and grandparents in particular, play in children's lives. The connection, shared activity and time together benefits both grandchildren and grandparents. Children bring love, energy, optimism, laughter, activity, youthfulness and purpose to their grandparents. Grandparents provide maturity, knowledge, stability and unconditional love to their grandchildren. Although it is a two-way street, my focus here is more on what your parents can do, as grandparents, to help your children and your family thrive.

❋ **Holder of collected wisdom.** Grandparents hold the collected wisdom and values of their generation and make it available, to be passed on as a guide or yardstick, to later generations. It may be crucial for children or young teenagers to experience a broader set of values than you

Formalising childcare agreements

Even though most grandparents will tell you that they get more out of looking after their grandchildren than they put into it, there is always the potential for any childcare arrangement to turn sour and for resentment or recriminations to emerge about the style or quality of the care.

Without honest, open and constant communication about the care-giving expectations each of you has, the most enthusiastic grandparent could come to regret saying yes to childcare. The most grateful parents may begin to make unreasonable demands. And the cutest grandchild may become too much for a grandparent to handle. To counteract this, it is worth formalising the agreement with your parent(s) if they are going to be a regular or long-term carer for your child. When this agreement has been finalised, it is worth reviewing it regularly. I suggest that you make explicit agreements about the following:

might have. Their grandparents can describe those values with a personal influence. That personal influence may be more supportive and helpful to your child than the wider cultural influences from society in general.

* **Historian.** Grandparents provide a unique link to the cultural and familial past for children. The tales they can tell about their own childhoods and their own families of origin enable children to feel connected to a sense of place and community. Even when your family lives in a different country from the one in which your parents were reared, there are aspects of your own history that have probably been influenced by theirs. Their experiences in a society that may have been markedly different from our own show

* Payment or not (about 20 per cent of grandparent carers are paid and some may need the money to supplement pensions)
* The times during which childcare is needed (including your commitment to drop/pick-up or return home on time)
* Where the childcare is to happen (including if you are happy for your parent(s) to run errands or visit others with your children in tow)
* The style of caring that you want and expect to be used (discuss this long and hard if necessary to be sure that you have common ground and that you are happy with everything)
* Any other jobs or commitments (like housework or feeding pets – don't assume that your mother or father will do everything that you would while caring for your child)
* A 'get-out clause' (agree to review the arrangements regularly so that both you and your parents have a no-blame opt-out if things don't seem to be working).

children how society and culture have changed, either for the better or for the worse.

* **Mentor.** Grandparents, typically, don't have to exercise control over your children in the same way as you do. This means that they can teach, share skills and talents, provide advice and listen to their grandchildren without being compromised by having to be the primary disciplinarian. They have a real opportunity to nurture their grandchildren and can be powerful role models in areas such as hard work or family loyalty. Children will often talk and listen to their grandparents in a way that is different from how they interact with other adults, giving grandparents a unique opportunity to guide and shape their lives.

❋ **Playmate.** Grandparents often have time to just be with children, with no agenda other than to hang out or play. When children can have fun with their grandparents, it can help them develop positive associations with ageing and older adults. Not that every grandparent is necessarily old when they inherit the job, but they do age!

❋ **Direct care-giver.** Many parents rely on their own parents for childcare at various stages in, or even throughout, their children's lives. They feel reassured that someone related to their child will be caring for them, since the grandparents will have a strong emotional commitment to the task.

Making it easy for grandparents to be connected to your thriving family

Assuming that your relationship with your parents is positive, you will want to facilitate their involvement in your family. However, do bear in mind that not all grandparents are itching to be that active in their role.

It is important to gauge the level of interest your parents show in being involved. You may already have seen their initial excitement about a baby's arrival wane as the baby became an active toddler or wilful pre-schooler. Your parents' energy levels, as they grow older, may not have kept pace with your expanding family and, correspondingly, they may have pulled back. While this may have seemed hurtful to you, it is quite a natural evolution. As grandchildren and grandparents age, their relationship can change.

Some grandparents may slow down as grandchildren grow up. Others may show more interest in older grandchildren, whom they find easier to take out or do things with. Similarly, small children have lots of time to just be with grandparents, while older ones may have busy schedules in which hanging out with Granny and Granddad may not feature very prominently.

Another block to including your parents may be their own availability. Not all grandparents fit the stereotype of the quiet, reserved and somewhat sedentary older person. Your parents may have their own busy and active lives, either continuing to work or as proactive retirees. Sometimes if we push too hard for our parents to be active in the lives of their grandchildren, their resentment may disrupt an otherwise positive relationship between them and their grandchild.

Think about where you meet your parents. When whole families descend on grandparents, they can feel beleaguered and become worn out quickly. Sometimes a neutral venue (like a walk in the park or a trip to a playground) or even your own home may make for a less stressful get-together.

The single biggest factor in the quality of your children's relationship with your parents is often your own relationship with them. Having a child can bring you closer to your own parents as you now share the experience of being a parent. On the other hand, if you have very different views about how to bring up children, this may give rise to serious friction between you.

Ironically, you and your parents probably both have the best interests of your children at heart, even if you don't see eye to eye on the best way to achieve them. It can be hard to make time to be with your parents if you feel tense, anxious or frustrated in their company. But, whatever your own experiences with your parents, your children may have an entirely different, more successful and fulfilling relationship with them. Even if it sticks in your craw a little, try to make space for them to develop their own relationship with your parents, unburdened by your history.

Ways to connect with grandparents who live far away

* Use the old-fashioned postal service to exchange photos, drawings and short notes as this may be easier for your parents, and envelopes dropping through the letterbox still excite children.

* Encourage your parents to use email and text messages to stay in touch with older children.
* Use the telephone but remember that your small children may not have much to say or may not want to be interrupted in their play.
* Keep your parents up-to-date about your child's interests and activities to help their conversations along, whether by phone, email or writing.
* Ask your parents to make audio books of your small children's favourite stories as an alternative to live bedtime stories or to fill in the gaps during the day.
* Use online social networking to its full advantage by creating a family profile that your parents can link into and contribute to, perhaps getting your older children to show their grandparents how it works when you do get to visit.

Acknowledgements

I would like to thank Ciara Considine, my editor in Hachette, for helping me to crack this book. Because of the many revisions, I think it finally represents what I really feel and believe about thriving families. I would also like to thank the many other people at Hachette who have been involved in the production of the book to the standard that you see it today.

I would like to thank my parents, Michael and Geraldine, who have given me the solid base that has allowed me to grow to be the man I am, with the beliefs that I hold.

I would like to thank Noel Kelly and Niamh Kirwan of NK Management for looking after all of my business affairs and keeping me solvent while I worked on the book. I want to mention special thanks to Niamh for her 're-focusing' chats, also known in text parlance as KUTA chats.

My biggest and most heartfelt appreciation goes to my family. Ironically, I haven't been very available to them to help them thrive while I have been squirrelled away writing. But they are a patient, warm and loving bunch. Conall, Megan and Éanna, yet again, are owed a debt of my time and my attention. Thank you for all of your co-operation and your occasional quiet games while I wrote. I love each of you dearly. Thank you.

My wife has kept our family thriving over the duration of my writing – emotionally, practically and psychologically. She will deny it, and perhaps say it was 'just what you have to do'. But I will not let her shrug off, or minimise, the huge commitment that she has shown to me, our family and this book. Michèle is a remarkable woman and a thoughtful, kind, respectful, honest, warm, loving, trustworthy and intensely responsible mother and wife. If our family thrives it is because she works hard to make it so. Thank you isn't really enough but it has to do. Thank you.